Keto for

Women

Over 50

JULIA CHRISTEN

OTHER BOOKS BY JULIA CHRISTEN

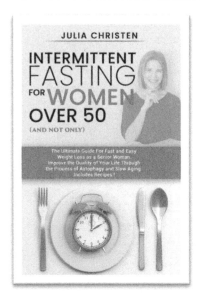

The Ultimate Guide For Fast and Easy Weight Loss as Senior Woman.
Improve the Quality of Your Life Through the Process of Autophagy and Slow Aging. Include Recipes!

Find it on Kindle Store
CLICK HERE

TABLE OF CONTENTS

Introduction

The following chapters will discuss exactly how easy it is to lose weight and maintain a healthy weight even after age fifty. The old saying is that age is just a number, and in most cases, it is, but women who are past age fifty know that this old saying is not exactly true. Once the woman has reached age fifty, her body goes through changes that are perfectly normal and perfectly aggravating at the same time! But this is an exciting time for a woman to be alive. This time is the time when many women finally come into their own space and begin to live life for themselves and what better way to do that than by taking control of your body and your health?

This book has all the answers you need to help you to do all of that. Once you understand the changes your body is going through and how to address these changes, you will begin to live the full, rich life that you deserve to live. Health and beauty begin on the inside, and this book will show you exactly how to get started on the changes that will carry you through the next chapter of your life.

There are plenty of books on this subject on the market, thanks again for choosing this one! Every effort was made to ensure it is full of as much useful information as possible, and please enjoy!

Chapter One

WHAT IS THE KETOGENIC DIET?

As far back as the ancient physicians in Greece, we have been told that healthy weight can easily be maintained by restricting the intake of calories from food. For centuries people fasted to treat various illnesses, particularly epilepsy. In the early twentieth century, doctors began experimenting with fasting as a way to control the effects of epilepsy, in the days before medications were introduced. It was found that people who subscribed to the 'water diet' had fewer seizures and were sometimes considered 'cured.' As you can probably guess the water diet consisted of water. And while people did enjoy a respite from seizures it is difficult to maintain a healthy lifestyle while consuming a diet made up of only water.

But this was an exciting time for medical discoveries as patients and physicians alike were beginning to wonder exactly what made the bodywork the way it did. An endocrinologist discovered that people who lived on the water diet secreted three compounds from their livers that were water-soluble, meaning they were flushed away by water. These three compounds together were called 'ketones.'

Since it was impossible to live on water for the remainder of a person's life, doctors began experimenting with different combinations of food so that their epileptic patients could eat.

They discovered that a diet that was lower in carbohydrates and rich in fats with a good amount of protein would produce the same epilepsy-free results that the water diet did. Patients could consume a diet of specific foods that mimicked the effect of fasting on their bodies. Eating more fat and removing sugar from the diet caused the liver to release the ketones that the body would then use for energy. Physicians had already concluded that the ketones the body was releasing were the main cause of epileptic seizures and since these were also released by the liver on a high-fat low carb diet, they named this diet the ketogenic diet.

So, physicians used this diet with great success on children and adults who had epilepsy. Seizures lessened or stopped altogether, and people were able to resume a normal life. But then doctors began noticing that people who followed the keto diet, the children especially, were displaying other changes in their bodies that went beyond the cessation of seizures. These people lost weight and were more active. They slept better at night and were more alert during the day. The children especially were easier to discipline and much less irritable than before.

But eventually, anticonvulsant drugs were invented that allowed people with epilepsy to take medication and be free from the restrictions of the dietary plan. This reversal of thought was during a time when refrigeration was still not widely used so that following the constraints of the keto diet may have been difficult for many people. And taking a pill was so much easier. So, the keto diet was no longer taught in medical school and generally fell out of favor with most doctors until a prominent event in the latter part of the twentieth century that changed the way people looked at keto and brought it into the modern world.

At that time a television producer and his wife were looking for something to help their young son who suffered from severe seizures. Even strong medications would not control the child's seizures that would often come one after the other. While doing internet research, his parents stumbled over a description of the ketogenic diet, which would eventually revolutionize their lives. When they started their young son on the keto diet, his seizures virtually vanished, and he was finally able to enjoy life as a normal little boy. A made-for-tv movie soon followed, and the world was once again in love with the keto diet.

But even with its success in treating epilepsy, the keto diet would not have been thought of so favorably if it did not help people to achieve and maintain a normal healthy weight. And while the keto diet itself is relatively new, this style of eating has been around since the time of early man. Hunting and gathering was a way of life for our ancient ancestors. They hunted meat and gathered plants and berries as they traveled from place to place hunting meat. And no part of the meat was wasted, which meant that early man also ate the fat part of the meat along with the lean part. As each generation has moved less and relied on processed foods more, we have gradually become more obese and less healthy.

Enter the keto diet. Following the keto diet relies on a heavy intake of fats, a moderate intake of protein, and a low intake of carbohydrates to achieve weight loss and later to maintain a healthy weight. The main function of the keto diet is to put your body into a state of ketosis which will then cause your body to produce ketones that your body will use for energy instead of using the sugar from the foods that you consume. A high carbohydrate diet will repress the ability of the body to produce ketones, and the excess sugar gets stored as fat.

When you eat the food that you consume goes into your stomach where acids and enzymes mix with the chewed food and help to break it down into even smaller particles. When your meal leaves your stomach, it has been liquified for easier passage into and through the small intestine. In the small intestine, the body completes the job of digesting your food and begins to move it into your bloodstream to other parts of the body. While your gall bladder produces bile to help digest your food and your liver stores nutrients and filters out toxins, your pancreas is perhaps the next most important organ in the food use process. The pancreas is the main organ in your body that helps to regulate your blood sugar levels through its production of insulin.

The hormone insulin is made by the pancreas to help your body use glucose (sugar) from the food that you eat for energy. While the body needs this sugar for energy the molecules of sugar do not pass into the cells by themselves. They need to attach to molecules of insulin in order to be able to enter the cells. When you consume food your blood sugar level rises and this triggers the pancreas to release insulin to help carry the sugar into the cells so that the cells can use the sugar for energy. The problem arises when people either eat too much food overall or they eat too many simple carbs that will turn into sugar in the body. When this happens, the body receives too many signals too often for increasing the level of insulin. Eventually, the cells will stop reacting to insulin because they are full of glucose and have no room for more. Then the excess glucose is stored in the body as excess body fat. When this happens you now have two overwhelming problems, insulin resistance, and obesity.

Many older women have a problem with excess belly fat, and the reason for this is simple. Excess glucose is stored as fat in the body, and the body will search for the easiest place to dump this glucose.

The cavities of the midsection, around the internal organs in the abdomen, are the perfect place – in the opinion of the body – to dump off all of that excess sugar so it can turn into fat. The insulin turns the glucose into glycogen and stores it in your belly for possible future needs.

So, it is a known fact that eating more food than you really need for survival leads to obesity. By continuously overeating we train our bodies to think that they need food all day long, which simply is not true. Many cultures around the world discourage snacking between meals and those people tend to live long healthy lives. So, we keep overeating and then one day we realize that we have a body that is filled with little pockets of fat. You will need to rid your body of this excess fat by exercising regularly and consuming a healthy diet. And this is where the keto diet will be the most beneficial.

While we refer to keto as the 'keto diet' it should not really be thought of as a diet. No one should ever plan to live on a diet forever, as that implies restricting things and we do not like to deprive ourselves. Rather, keto should be thought of as a way of life that you will follow in order to make yourself be healthy and fit. When you live the keto way of life your body will start by breaking down excess fat and using these reserves for energy. This is what the body does naturally during times of starvation; it uses stored fat to fuel the body when new food sources are not readily available.

But won't any diet plan work for that purpose? No, not really. Remember that the woman's body naturally stores an extra bit of fat in case we get pregnant. We need to have enough energy in reserve to feed the growing baby. And this is exactly why a man and a woman will have drastically different results on the same diet. The man will lose weight while the woman probably won't and might even gain weight. When a man cuts calories his body turns to stored fat reserves. When a woman cuts calories her metabolism slows down.

The keto diet does not care if you are male or female because it works the same way on everybody. The keto diet restricts carb intake to a level that forces the liver to produce ketones that cause the body to burn stored fat for fuel. The liver naturally produces ketones, just not at the level that it does during ketosis. The liver stores glucose as glycogen and the body will fill up the liver before it fills up any other space in the body. When the body is deprived of substantial carbohydrate intake it turns to the glycogen in the liver to produce energy for the functions of the cells. Since the liver can only store about forty-eight hours with glycogen for energy it must then turn to outside sources like belly fat. When your liver is depleted of stored glycogen and begins to take stores from the body to metabolize for energy then you have entered the state of ketosis.

Do not confuse ketosis with ketoacidosis which is a harmful condition brought on as a result of Type 1 Diabetes.

Ketosis comes on anywhere from two days to one week after beginning the keto diet. This is the goal of the keto diet, to push your body into ketosis. Once you have reached a state of ketosis you will need to maintain the diet in order to remain in ketosis. Getting into ketosis is the worst side effect of the keto diet but once you get past the initial stage you will not regret your decision. Ketosis is often referred to as keto flu because the symptoms feel much like you have viral flu. The symptoms of beginning ketosis are varied:

- Sleep disturbances
- Exhaustion

- Headaches
- Irritability and moodiness
- Bad breath
- Weakness during exercise and after
- Constipation
- Bloating
- Cravings for sugary foods
- Temporary loss of libido
- Diarrhea

The bad breath of ketosis is caused by waste products being eliminated from your body. These waste products are stored in fat cells and need to be eliminated as the fat cells are eliminated. Your body will eliminate waste through your breath, your sweat, or through defecation or urination.

You might naturally feel deprived of sugary treats when you begin the keto diet. We all love a good glazed doughnut or a huge bowl of cake and ice cream and we miss these when they are gone. Just remember they are not gone forever and there are plenty of satisfying dessert options on the keto diet. You will crave carbs because they taste good, but you will be consuming enough foods so that you will not need the carbs to make up for the caloric intake. And decreasing carb intake may lead to a decrease in your ability to get a good night's sleep. Consuming carbs causes the brain to release hormones melatonin and serotonin which are the hormones that make you sleepy and happy respectively. Eventually, the keto diet will teach your body to release hormones at the proper times but in the meantime try to keep a consistent sleep schedule even on your days off.

Some people will experience bloating, constipation, or diarrhea when beginning the keto diet. Food affects all people differently. Diarrhea comes from the increase in fats in your diet. The bloating is from the body releasing toxins from the stored fats that are being digested. Constipation may also go along with increased urination. Fat cells are the primary sources of water storage in your body. When you begin eliminating fat cells the excess water leaves your body in the form of perspiration or urination, leaving very little for the bowels to use for defecation. And less water in your body may lead to feelings of fatigue or muscle weakness.

Moodiness and irritability come from the fact that you are now consuming fewer carbs than before. Carbs almost immediately turn into sugar when they are consumed, and this is true whether the carb is a honey bun or a potato. The body does not care about the difference in healthy or unhealthy food, it just cares that food is coming in. Excess levels of sugar in the blood cause the body to release the hormones dopamine and serotonin which make you calm and happy. This is also why people often fall asleep after consuming a meal that is full of carbs. Removing these foods means that the brain will not signal the release of these hormones and you might feel irritable or moody for a few days.

High-fat diets will increase the level of estrogen in the woman's body because estrogen is stored in fat. So, the more estrogen you have in your body the higher your desire for sexual activity will be, and this is often lost during the first days of ketosis as all of those stored fat cells begin to disappear. When the body has eliminated enough stored fat and has begun functioning at a proper level then the hormone levels will balance themselves out, the estrogen production will return to normal, and your sex drive will reappear.

While these all might seem like good reasons to avoid the keto diet altogether, remember that these side effects are temporary and the beneficial effects of the keto diet are permanent. There are things that you can do to combat the effects of the keto flu and the beginning of ketosis to help you get through this period:

- Drink plenty of water to stay hydrated
- Add sea salt to your water to help ease muscle cramps. Lemon juice will help mask the saltiness
- Engage in gentle exercises like walking, bicycling, or swimming
- Chew gum or suck mints that are sugar-free
- Get a regularly scheduled seven to nine hours of sleep every night

Focusing on the positive benefits of the keto diet may also help you get through ketosis. The keto diet will naturally promote weight loss and assist you with managing your weight. You can easily incorporate the keto diet into your regular lifestyle. Fats and proteins will make you feel full for a longer time so you will eventually consume less food. Food cravings will disappear and hunger will be eliminated. There is really no need to count calories on the keto diet unless you are going for a specific weight loss goal. Keto will not slow down your metabolism so you will continue to lose weight even after the first few weeks on the diet. You will feel more energetic and will be able to better focus on everyday tasks. Your muscles will become stronger and leaner.

Keto flu fades away and you are left with the positive side effect of the keto diet which will last your entire lifetime. All bodies are different and you may not see the same results that your neighbor might enjoy on the same diet plan. But follow the diet, eat the right foods, and you will be successful.

Chapter Two

CHANGES IN YOUR BODY AFTER AGE 50

If you have reached age fifty, then you should congratulate yourself. You have been through school, teen years, relationships, children, and most importantly the changing of your body. You might be looking at your body and asking it exactly what happened during the last few years. Some things you have not been able to control, like hereditary medical issues and the ravage that time puts on our bodies. Accidents and illnesses are also beyond our control. But you can begin now to understand the changes in your body and make plans to reduce or eliminate as many of the negative changes as you possibly can.

The first thing that will probably happen to you is the onset of menopause. The most notable thing about menopause is that your monthly periods will stop – forever! Menopause is the biggest single change that your body will ever experience besides puberty. Menopause can lead to belly fat, weight gain, and osteoporosis. It is a natural occurrence in the life of every woman, caused by the body making less of the hormones estrogen and progesterone.

Estrogens (there are more than one) is the name for the group of sex-related hormones that make women be women. They cause and promote the initial development and further maintenance of female characteristics in the human body. Estrogens are what gave you breasts, hair in the right places, the ability to reproduce, and your monthly cycle. Estrogen is the hormone that does all of the long-term work in maintaining femininity. Progesterone has one purpose in the woman's body, and that is to implant the egg in the uterus and keep her pregnant until it is time to deliver the baby.

In women, estrogen is crucial to becoming and remaining womanly. In the ovaries, it stimulates the growth of eggs for reproduction. It causes the vagina to grow to a proper adult size. Estrogen promotes the healthy growth of the fallopian tubes and the uterus. And it causes your breasts to grow and to fill with milk when the baby is coming. Estrogen is also responsible for making women store some excess fat around their thighs and hips. This weight storage is nature's way of ensuring that the baby will have nutrition during times of famine.

One of the forms of estrogen dramatically decreases in production after menopause, and this form helps women to regulate the rate of their metabolism and how fast they gain weight. After menopause women tend to gain more weight in their middle area of the body, in the abdomen. This fat collects around the organs and is known as visceral fat. Besides being unattractive visceral fat is also dangerous, because it has been linked to some cancers, heart disease, stroke, and diabetes.

But a lack of estrogen is not the only reason women tend to gain weight after age fifty. Besides a lack of estrogen, the biggest single reason that women over fifty gain weight is lifestyle changes. They are no longer running children to activities; so many women move less after fifty. And sometimes they move less because their joints have begun to ache. Stiffness begins to set in, especially in the morning when rolling out of bed suddenly becomes a chore. Many continue to cook large meals and have difficulty scaling back to cooking for just one or two people, and someone needs to eat that food. And some women still feel that life ends when the children leave so they might as well just indulge a little.

But all of this indulging and relaxing leads to loss of muscle strength, loss of flexibility, and increased belly fat, which in turn leads to even more problems. It also leads to an increase in osteoporosis. The lack of estrogen is the leading cause of osteoporosis, which translates literally to the porous bone. The bones in the body, particularly the long bones of the arms and the legs, become more porous as the quality and density of the bone is reduced. Bones will continue to regrow and refresh themselves all of your life, but in osteoporosis, the bone is deteriorating faster than new growth can replace it.

Estrogen helps to decrease overall cholesterol levels in young women which is why women sometimes remain healthy even when they don't take the time to eat healthy meals. All of these changes after fifty and the arrival of menopause because suddenly the estrogen levels drop dramatically. This increase in cholesterol in the body can lead to strokes and heart attacks. Cholesterol is a substance that occurs naturally in your body and is made by the liver. Cholesterol in your body also comes from the foods that you eat. The two kinds that your doctor will measure with a blood test are high-density lipoprotein (HDL) and low-density lipoprotein (LDL). The two numbers together make up your total cholesterol number. Estrogen promotes HDL and depresses LDL, so a lack of estrogen will allow for a higher LDL number.

HDL is the type of cholesterol known as the good type because it removes excess amounts of cholesterol from your arteries and then carries it to the liver where it can be metabolized and removed from the body during waste removal. LDL is the bad form of cholesterol because it likes to sit in your arteries and form deposits known as plaque. It is possible to have a high total cholesterol number and still be considered healthy if the number is high because the HDL is high and the LDL is low. This means that your body is doing the right thing and the good cholesterol is eliminating the bad cholesterol.

When LDL clumps in the arteries and forms plaques it causes hardening of the arteries. Blood will not flow very well through stiff arteries. Your heart will need to work harder to push the blood through your body. And if you have gained a significant amount of weight your body has created new arteries to supply blood flow to this increased part of you. This will also make the heart work harder than it needs to. And if plaque builds up in the arteries that are connected to the heart those arteries can become clogged which results in coronary artery disease. This can cause a heart attack if a piece of plaque breaks loose and cuts off the steady flow of blood to the muscles of the heart. If this happens in the arteries that lead to the brain it can cause a stroke.

Too much cholesterol has also been found in the brains of people who suffered from Alzheimer's disease. And an excessive amount of cholesterol can cause gallstones, which women are naturally at a higher risk of anyway.

You may have noticed that you seem to be losing control of your bladder function, or that laughing or sneezing makes you dribble a bit. This is also a normal effect of aging because the muscles just are not as strong as they used to be. Also, the excess weight pressing down on the bladder does not help the situation.

While it is impossible to stop the process of aging there are things every woman can do to slow the process and help her body remain healthy far into the future. One of the most important ways women can do this is to maintain a healthy weight, which is what makes the keto diet is so important to all women and especially to those over age fifty.

Chapter Three

USING KETO TO CONTROL OR PREVENT AGE-RELATED CONDITIONS

E veryone gradually gets older. It is an undeniable fact of life. But even though we are aging all of the time, we do not need to be old, not yet anyway. It is possible to be an active, vibrant woman at fifty and beyond if you make some smart choices and take care of yourself. And deciding to follow the keto way of life is the smartest choice you could have made. The keto diet isn't just good for weight loss, although that is probably its most important and noticeable feature. The keto diet gives so much more to your body while it is helping you to lose and then maintain your weight.

The keto diet will result in increased brain function and the ability to focus. The brain normally uses sugar to fuel its processes, but the consumption of sugar has its own problems. The brain can easily switch to using ketones for fuel and energy. Remember that ketones are the by-product of ketosis that makes you burn fat. And the keto diet was used by doctors to control seizures in patients long before medications were invented. The exact way this works is still not completely understood, but researchers believe it has something to do with the neurons stabilizing as excess sugar is removed from the diet and hormones are better regulated. Patients

17

with Alzheimer's disease have been seen to have increased cognitive function and enhanced memory when they consume a keto diet. And these same changes in the chemical makeup of the brain can lead to fewer migraines overall and less severe migraines.

When the keto diet helps you to lose weight, it also helps you to reduce your risk of cardiovascular disease. These diseases include anything that pertains to the cardiovascular system, which means heart attacks, strokes, plaque formations, peripheral artery disease, blood clots, and high blood pressure. Plaque buildups, which are caused by excess weight and cholesterol, lead to a condition known as atherosclerosis. The plaque will gather in the arteries and form clogs that narrow the artery and restrict the flow of blood. The plaque is formed from fat cells, waste products, and calcium deposits that are found floating in the blood. When you lose weight and decrease the amount of fat and cholesterol in the body there will be less to accumulate in the arteries and the blood will naturally flow better with less restriction.

Being overweight can cause high blood pressure. When the doctor measures the force of your blood pressure as it moves through your arteries, he is measuring your blood pressure. If you are overweight your heart will need to push the blood harder to get it through the increased lengths of arteries it had to create in order to feed your cells. And if there is a buildup of plaque in the arteries then the heart will need to push the blood harder to get it past the blockage. This, in turn, creates thin spots in the arteries which is a good place for plaque to build up. Since this condition comes on gradually over the course of years as you slowly gain weight it gives off no immediate symptoms and that is why it is often referred to as the silent killer. Strokes and heart attacks are caused by unchecked high blood pressure.

The single most important way to control high blood pressure is to control your weight. You can't change the family history but you can control your weight and your lifestyle. Since high blood pressure is caused by the heart needing to work harder than the act reducing the strain on the heart will cause it to work less strenuously in bad ways. Losing weight and maintaining a healthy weight will ease the strain on your heart. If the blood pressure is not pumping too high then it will not cause weak spots in your arteries. If there are no weak spots then there is no place for plaque to collect. And if there is no excess fat or cholesterol in the blood there will be no plaque formations to collect in the blood.

A diet that is high in saturated fats is a risk factor for heart disease. While keto is a high-fat diet it is high in monounsaturated fats. Polyunsaturated and monounsaturated fats are good for you while trans fats and saturated fats are not. Mono – and polyunsaturated fats are the good fats that are found in fatty fish like salmon and in certain plants like avocados, olives, and certain seeds and nuts that are all staples of the keto diet. Saturated fats and trans fats are found in breaded deep-fried foods, baked goods, processed foods, and pre-packaged snack foods like popcorn. When your doctor measures your LDL and HDL he also measures your level of triglycerides, which is a type of fat that is found floating in the bloodstream and that is responsible for elevating the risk of heart attacks, especially in women over fifty. Reducing the number of saturated fats and trans fats that you consume will automatically reduce the amounts of triglycerides floating in your blood.

Inflammation is a part of life, especially for women over the age of fifty. There are good kinds of inflammation, such as when white blood cells rush to a particular body area to kill an infection. But mostly older women are plagued by the bad forms of inflammation which make your joints swell and cause early morning stiffness.

19

Carrying too much weight on your body will cause inflammation and pain in the joints, especially in the lower part of the body where the weight-bearing joints like the knees and the hips are located. When a joint feels pain it sends a signal to the brain that there is a pain, and the body sends cells to combat that pain. The helper cells don't know there really isn't anything wrong but they come prepared to fight and this causes inflammation around the joint. One extra pound of excess weight will put four pounds of pressure on the knee joints. Losing weight will help to eliminate inflammation in the body. And cutting down on the intake of carbs will help to lessen the amount of inflammation in the body because carbs cause inflammation. Decreasing the inflammation in your body will also help to eliminate acne, eczema, arthritis, psoriasis, and irritable bowel syndrome.

Adopting the keto way of life will also help to eliminate problems with the kidneys and improve their function. Kidney stones and gout are caused mainly by the elevation of certain chemicals in the urine that helps to create uric acid which is what we eliminate in the bathroom. The excess consumption of carbohydrates and sugar will lead to a buildup of calcium and phosphorus in your urine. This buildup of excess chemicals can cause kidney stones and gout. When your ketones begin to raise the acid in your urine will briefly increase as your body begins to eliminate all of the waste products from the fats that are being metabolized, but after that, the level will decrease and will remain lower than before as long as you are on the keto diet.

Eating a diet that is high carb can eventually cause problems with your gallbladder including gallstones. These stones are little deposits of hardened fluid that get trapped in your gallbladder and cause great pain. The gallbladder is built to release bile into the small intestine to help digest the food that you eat. When the liver produces more cholesterol than your gallbladder can produce bile to digest, the excess cholesterol forms stones in the gallbladder. Eating a low carb diet will eliminate much of the excess cholesterol that your liver produces and the high fat of the keto diet will help the gallbladder to cleanse itself.

Vegetables that grow in the ground, grain-based foods, processed foods, and sugary foods all contribute to heartburn and acid reflux by raising the level of acid in the stomach. There is a band of muscles that is wound tightly around the bottom of your esophagus, the muscular tube that takes food from your mouth to your stomach. This band of muscles is called the esophageal sphincter. It will relax just enough to let food pass into the stomach when it is healthy. But a constant diet of the wrong kinds of foods will increase the stomach acid, which in turn washes over this sphincter and eventually weakens it, which allows stomach acid to flow backward and up into the esophagus. Eating the low carb keto diet will improve the acid reflux symptoms and will help to relieve the inflammation of the esophagus and the stomach.

The best overall benefit of the keto lifestyle is the fact that it will lower your overall weight, which will have a positive effect on your entire body. Lower weight will mean freedom from the effects of obesity which can help to get rid of metabolic syndrome and Type 2 Diabetes. The condition known as Metabolic Syndrome happens when the body becomes resistant to insulin and the insulin your body produces is no recognized by the cells in your body. This is what causes the body to store your excess blood sugar as fat in your body, especially around the area of the stomach. When you begin the keto diet and enter ketosis the body will be forced to use these fat stores for energy and the body's production of insulin will be returned to normal. The amount of protein in the diet will help your muscles keep their strength and tone and not begin to wither as so often happens in older women.

Following the keto diet will mean that you will eat less food but it will be more filling and more nutritious. When you eat fats and proteins instead of carbs you will feel fuller much longer with less food. Lowering your caloric intake will help you lose weight and less weight will make you healthier. It will also slash your risk of developing certain diseases and will minimize the effects of others. These are the life improvements that the keto lifestyle has to offer you.

Chapter Four

FOOD LIST FOR KETO EATING

I f you have done any reading on the keto diet or heard other people talking about it. If so, you may have heard the term 'macros.' It sounds like a magical, mystical term that goes along with this new magical diet plan. People who have lived the keto lifestyle for a while love to share their knowledge, and some of it is very good. But there is a huge difference of opinion when it comes to the macros.

Macros are nothing more than a shortened version of the word macronutrient. A macronutrient is a component of the food that you use to fuel your body. In other words, a macro is a fat, protein, or carbohydrate. In the opinion of some people, you need to track your macros in order to make certain that you are getting the correct balance of nutrients. And some people feel that you do not need to track your macros as long as you correctly follow the guidelines for the keto diet that pertain to avoiding carbs and eating a high-fat diet.

On a standard keto diet, you will consume a diet that is five percent carbohydrates, twenty to twenty-five percent proteins, and seventy-five percent fats. If you are counting your macros then you will need to decide how many calories you want to consume in one day, and then you will need to multiply your food percentages by your total calories to see how many calories of each macro you can eat in one day. The calculation would look something like this:

2000 calorie diet

2000 x 5% carbs = 100 grams of carbs

2000 x 20% proteins = 400 grams of proteins

2000 x 75% fats = 1500 grams of fats

The key is in knowing exactly what is in your food. So, on the keto diet, you will either read a lot of food labels or you will be making most of your food from scratch. The number of calories that you choose to consume will depend on many factors such as your height, activity level, and how much weight you want to lose.

You will notice that the ratio of carbs on the keto diet is very low. There are good reasons for this. Carbs turn directly to sugar when they are consumed, and the type of carb does not matter; eventually, they all will produce some amount of sugar in your body during digestion. A complex carb, such as a potato or a beet, will take longer to digest and will make less sugar than a sweet roll or a slice of bread, but they all turn out the same way. Also, there is no real essential carbohydrate. There are essential amino acids (proteins) and fatty acids (fats), but there are no carbs that you must eat in order to maintain a healthy lifestyle.

When you are reading food labels or recipe information there is a particular way to know how many net carbs are in the food that you are eating. So look on a nutrition label and find the line that says 'total carbs.' Then find the line that says 'fiber.' Fiber is considered a carb but it does not count toward your total carb intake because fiber passes through your body as waste because it is not digestible. So, you will subtract the amount of fiber from the total carbs number to decide your net carb count, like this:

17 grams of carbs – 5 grams of fiber = 12 grams of net carbs

Net carbs are the starches and sugars that are leftover when the fiber count is removed. This is the number that you will count toward your daily allowance of carbs. You will need to know which foods are low in carbs and which ones you should eat rarely or never. And when you are looking for those added carbs on your food labels you want to look for glucose, sucrose, dextrose, fructose, galactose, maltose, cellulose, dextrin, glycogen, and any word that ends in saccharide. Words to look for that will alert you to the added presence of added sugar are cane sugar, corn sugar, brown sugar, confectioner's sugar, beet sugar, beetroot, grape sugar, dextrose, fruit sugar, levulose, maltose, malt sugar, lactose, milk sugar, invert sugar, maple sugar, and saccharose.

When you think about the foods that are allowed on the keto diet you might begin to think that the keto diet is the most restrictive diet you have ever seen. In one way it is because you will not be allowed to eat those sugary treats you might be so fond of. But there are plenty of tasty carbs that are allowed on the keto diet, and they are carbs that are good for your body. Some will say that everything that you eat should be organic and fresh. Meat should be grass-fed or free-range, eggs should come from free-range chickens and cheese should be made from the milk of grass-fed cows. While this is nice it just isn't necessary. Organic food is usually more expensive than similar non-organic food and it may not be easily available where you live. And not all food should be purchased fresh. If you live in a city with open-air markets or you like going to the grocery store several times each week then you can buy all of your food fresh. But for most people, this just is not realistic. Canned or frozen food is perfectly fine for the purposes of the keto diet. You will lose weight and eat good food on the keto diet whether it is organic or the same stuff everyone else eats.

So, what are you allowed to eat on the keto diet? Well, there are actually a great many foods that are allowed for keto dieters. You will eat meat, fish, seafood, vegetables, dairy items, fruits, and high-quality fats.

Fish and seafood are rich in the B vitamins as well as selenium and potassium. They are also rich in protein and carbohydrate-free. They are also great sources of Omega-3 fats which will help to increase your sensitivity to insulin and will help to lower the levels of sugar in your blood. You should eat fish and seafood at least two to three times each week.

Nutritional information per three-ounce serving without skin:

FOOD	CALORIES	PROTEIN	CARBS	FAT
Catfish	120	19	0	5
Clams, steamed, 12	120	22	4	2
Cod	90	19	0	1
Flounder	100	20	0	1
Haddock	90	20	0	1
Lobster	100	20	1	1
Mackerel	190	21	0	12
Perch	100	20	0	2
Orange Roughy	70	16	0	1
Oysters, steamed, 12	120	12	7	4
Pollock	100	21	0	1
Rainbow Trout	130	22	0	4
Salmon	150	22	0	7
Scallops, broiled, 14 small	150	29	2	1
Shrimp	110	22	0	2

Sole	100	21	0	1
Whiting	100	19	0	1

Meat and poultry are stapling items on the keto diet and excellent sources of protein. They are generally carb-free and are good sources of the B vitamins as well as the minerals zinc, selenium, and potassium. Bacon and sausage are processed meats that are allowed on the keto diet but they are sources of certain items that might raise your risk for cancer, so limit them whenever possible. Hot dogs and smoked sausage are also good choices but make sure to check the label and look for added sources of sugars or starches.

Here are the nutritional values for three-ounce servings of meats, poultry, and pork:

FOOD	CALORIES	PROTEIN	FAT	CARBS
Beef	220	27	12	0
Chicken, thigh	209	26	10.9	0
Chicken, breast	165	31	3.6	0
Turkey, breast	167	34	2	0
Hot dog, no bun	290	9	23	9
Smoked sausage	210	7	18	4
Pork, tenderloin	125	22	304	0
Pork, cutlet	239	34	10	0
Pork, ground	251	22	18	0
Bacon, one slice	37	3	3	0

The next category in which you will find keto-friendly foods is the dairy department. Certain dairy foods contain a good mix of fats, proteins, and carbs and they are also good sources of Vitamin B-12, calcium, and riboflavin. The nutritional values for the cheese in the following table are for one-ounce servings:

FOOD	CALORIES	CARBS	FATS	PROTEIN
Blue cheese	100	0.7	8.1	6

Brie	95	0.1	7.9	5.9
Cheddar	114	0.4	9.4	7
Cottage cheese	24	1	0.7	3.4
Cream cheese	97	1.2	9.7	1.7
Feta	75	1.2	9.7	1.7
Monterey Jack	106	0.2	8.6	6.9
Mozzarella	85	0.6	6.3	6.3
Parmesan	111	0.9	7.3	10
Swiss	108	1.5	7.9	7.6
Heavy cream, 2 Tbs.	104	0.8	11	0.6
Sour cream, 2 Tbs.	46	0.7	4.7	0.5
Greek yogurt	95	4	5	9
Egg, one	75	0.6	5	7

Vegetables will be your source of carbs and fiber in your diet. These nutritional values are for a one-cup serving unless otherwise noted:

Column1	Column2	Column3	Column4
FOOD	CARBS	FIBER	NET CARBS
Bell peppers	9	3	6
Broccoli	6	2	4
Asparagus	8	4	4
Mushrooms	2	1	1
Zucchini	4	1	3
Spinach, cooked	7	4	3
Spinach, raw	1	1	0
Avocados	13	10	3
Cauliflower	5	3	2
Green beans	10	4	6
Lettuce	2	1	1
Garlic, one cove	1	0.5	0.5
Kale	7	1	6
Cucumbers	4	1	3
Brussels Sprouts	6	2	4
Celery	3	2	1
Tomatoes	6	2	4

Radishes	4	2	2
Onions, one half cup	6	1	5
Eggplant	8	2	6
Cabbage	5	3	2
Artichokes	14	10	4

There are very few fruits that are allowed on the keto diet because the fruit is high in sugar. But the following fruits are allowed and these counts are for a half-cup serving:

FOOD	CARBS	FIBER	NET CARBS
Blackberries	6.9	3.8	3.1
Rhubarb	5.7	4	1.7
Star Fruit	4.4	1.8	2.6
Raspberries	7.3	4	3.3
Cantaloupe	6.8	1	5.8
Strawberries	5.7	1	4.7
Watermelon	6.4	1	5.4
Lemon	2.5	2	0.5
Lime	2.5	2	0.5

You should also stock up on the following food items. These are encouraged for use on the keto diet since some, like broth, will help you to curb hunger between meals and herbs and spices will add flavor to your food without adding carbs or calories. Just remember to look at the label for added starches and sugars:

Olive oil, coconut oil, avocado oil	Lard
Canned fish	Olives, green and black
Sauerkraut	Hot sauce

Flavored water additives, no sugar	Bottled water
Tea	Coffee
Club soda	Herbs and spices
Pork rinds (great for breading foods)	Mayonnaise, full fat
Mustard	Vinegar
Broth	Bouillon cubes

When you go food shopping only buy the things that you know you will eat. That may sound silly but some people will buy a portion of food they do not like just because it is listed on a diet plan. Don't do it! Buy the foods that you want to eat and leave the others for someone else. But also, don't be afraid to try foods you've never tried before or didn't like in the past. The adult you just might like radishes.

It is imperative that you get used to eating real food. Processes food has no place in the life of the keto dieter. Following the keto lifestyle will take more planning than any other diet or meal plan you may have tried, but it is totally worth the effort. Sometimes you might want to cook one large meal and divide it over several days of eating. Many recipes make great leftovers for tomorrow's lunch.

The keto diet does not mean giving up good food or the treats you once indulged in. It does mean making better food choices in order to improve your overall health and well-being. When you begin creating your own menus do not be afraid to experiment with different menu ideas and different ways of putting your food together. You will be pleasantly surprised at just how flexible and how good keto eating really is.

Chapter Five

EXERCISES TO ASSIST WITH QUALITY OF LIFE AFTER 50

The ways that you take care of your body and the ways you stay active will dictate your quality of life and how good you will look. If you do not take care of your body, you might be fifty years old and look like you are sixty-five years old. But if you do good things for your body you might be sixty-five years old and look like you are fifty years old. Age really is just a number. And even if you haven't been active in a long time, or ever, it is never too late to start on some sort of activity plan to increase the quality of your life.

I call it an activity plan because no one really wants to exercise, right? So, let's think of this as an activity plan or a workout routine, both of those are positive statements that say you care about your body and you want to fight the effects of growing older with everything you've got.

Once a woman crosses that fifty-year mark, she begins losing one percent of her muscle each year. But muscle tone and fiber do not need to be lost with aging. With a proper workout, you can continue to build new muscle and maintain what you already have until you are in your nineties. And some of the exercises that you do for your muscles will help you build strong bones. This is especially important for women because losing the estrogen supplies in our bodies will cause us to lose bone mass faster than men do. This is when we are really at risk for developing osteoporosis.

And regular physical activity will help you to avoid developing that middle-age spread around the abdomen or to lose it if you already have it. Activity will help you to maintain a proper weight for your height and build which in turn will help you to avoid many, if not all, of the age-related, obesity-related diseases such as cardiovascular diseases and diabetes.

Physical activity comes in four main types. Each one should be done at least once or twice a week to ensure your body is getting the right mix of activity. The four main types of activity are:

- Balance – Older people lose their sense of balance. It is easy for an older person to fall and break something, like a hip. When you engage in activities that help you to maintain your sense of balance will help reduce the risk that you might fall and suffer a permanent injury.

- Stretching – As we age our muscles begin to lose their elasticity. This is part of why rolling out of bed in the morning gets more difficult as we get older. Stretching activities will help you to improve and maintain your level of flexibility which will help you to avoid injuries to your joints and muscles.

- Cardiovascular/Aerobic – These are also called endurance activities because you should be able to maintain them for at least ten minutes at a time. This key here is to get your heart working faster and your breathing to be deeper. You should be working hard but still able to carry on a conversation. These activities will strengthen your heart and lungs which are, after all, very important muscles in your body.

- Strength training – We are not talking about bodybuilding, but if you want to go for it. This will include working out with resistance bands or lifting weights. Either activity will help to build muscle.

While there are four separate categories of exercise that does not mean that you need to keep them strictly separated because many activities will encompass work in more than one area. You can lift light weights while doing balance activities. Walking and swimming will build muscle strength and cardiovascular health. Yoga will improve balance and assist with building muscle strength and stretching. The key is to engage in seventy-five minutes of vigorous activity each week, or fifteen minutes five days each week; or you can get one hundred fifty minutes of moderate activity in five thirty-minute sessions each week.

And make sure that you design a plan that fits you. Remember that it is perfectly fine to change your routine as your needs change. Maybe, in the beginning, you will work on balance three days each week because you really need help with that. But after a few weeks, your balance has improved enough so that you can devote one of those days to strength training. This is your routine made just for you so make it work for you. And don't forget to get your doctor's okay before beginning any type of activity routine. He will most likely give you his blessings but it is always good to ask. He can also provide you with information on activities that are good for you personally.

One thing to note here, especially if you have not been active in a while, is not to begin a vigorous level of activity the same day you begin the keto diet. During the time your body is getting used to the diet and going through ketosis, you will not feel like indulging in a lot of extra activity and your workout routine will be doomed to failure. This journey is all about making you the best you possibly can so don't sabotage yourself in the first few weeks. If you really want to start your activities on day one of your diet then I recommend walking or bicycling. Either of these activities can be started slowly, so a gentle walk or bike around the neighborhood after dinner is a perfect activity.

If you can get out and join a class at a local senior center, YMCA, community college, or church then do that. You will meet new people, some in your age group, and you can all work together to create your new bodies. But taking a class will not be the best choice for everyone. So we have included some basic exercises that can be done in the privacy of your home to get you started on the new lean you.

STRETCHING – Stretching activities are so important for older adults. These activities will also help you to improve your balance because you might find yourself standing or reaching in new and different ways.

Quad stretch – This is a simple exercise that can be done at home. Hold onto a chair or your partner for balance assistance if you need it. Then with the opposite hand lift the foot on that side behind you. Pull upward gently you can feel the beginning of a stretch in the front of your leg. As people get older, they may lean forward for balance and this muscle, the quad, can become shorter and less efficient over time. Hold this position steady for at least thirty seconds and repeat on the other side.

Hamstring stretch – This activity can be done on the sofa, the bed, or on the floor. Lay one leg in front of you and point your toes to the ceiling. Slowly fold your body over until you feel a stretching in the back of your leg and hold it for thirty seconds. NOTE: if you have recently had a hip replacement check with your doctor before doing this one.

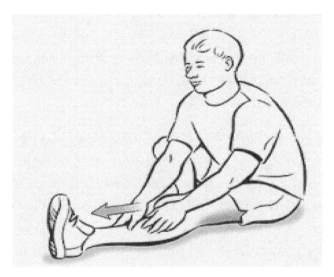

Calf stretch – Place your hands on the wall and step back with one foot. The back foot should be flat on the floor and the front knee should be slightly bent. Then lean forward toward the wall until you feel a stretch in your calf muscle. Hold it for thirty seconds and repeat on the other leg.

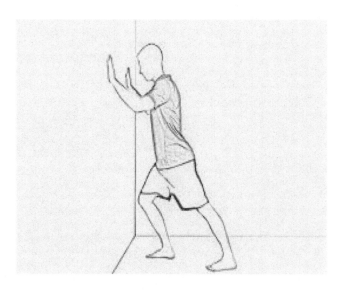

BALANCING – Balancing activities are so important for older adults to reduce the risk of falls. Tai Chi and Yoga are both excellent activities for assisting with better balance. You can find DVDs, routines online, or classes taught by certified instructors. Just remember to work with your body and your current level of ability and don't try to do an advanced routine if you have never mastered a beginner routine. You will just be setting yourself up for failure and we are here to succeed. And keep in mind that flexibility activities also help with the effects of arthritis. While you will want to explore the different types of yoga before making a decision on the one that is best for you, here is a yoga pose that anyone can do at home and helps to wake the whole body in the morning.

Mountain Pose – Stand straight with your feet together. Pull in your stomach muscles as tight as you can and let your shoulders relax. Keep your legs strong but do not lock your knees. Breathe deeply and regularly in and out for ten breaths.

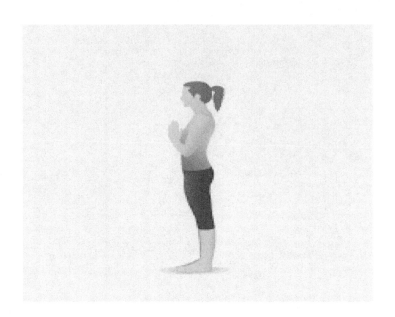

Strength Training – This activity is especially important for you to ensure you keep your muscles strong and healthy for the next phase of your life. You can do many strength training activities without weights, or for an extra challenge add some light hand weights.

Punching – This will strengthen your arms and shoulders and get your blood moving at the same time. Stand straight with your feet apart slightly wider than your shoulders. Keep your stomach firm. Punch straight out with one fist and then the other for at least twenty repetitions.

Squat – This activity is great for strengthening the bottom and the thighs. This will help you to sit down – not fall down – and be able to rise from a seated position with ease and grace. Stand with your feet as far apart as your hips are wide to provide a stable stance. Push your bottom backward as you bend your knees. Your knees should never go out front further than your toes, and try to keep your weight over your heels. If you feel more secure this activity can be done in front of a chair in case you lose your balance and inadvertently sit down.

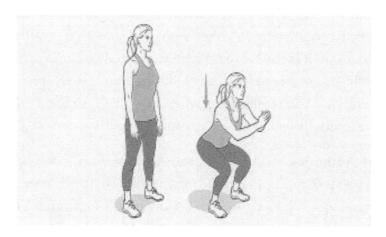

Bridge – Lie on your back with your knees bent and your feet as far apart as your hips. Keep your feet flat on the floor. Pull in your stomach and lift your hips to make a bridge of your back. Hold this pose for ten seconds and try to do at least ten.

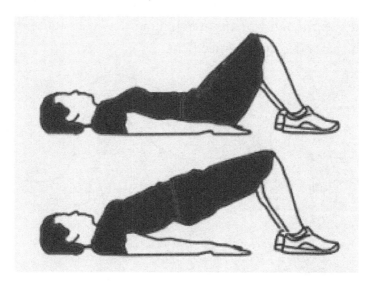

Cardiovascular/Aerobic – The purpose here is to engage in some activity that gets your heart pumping faster and your lungs expanding further. Swimming, walking, running, cycling, aerobics classes, dancing – all of these are great activities for getting the circulation going again. Just remember to begin slowly and pay attention to your body. In other words, if something hurts, stop. But make sure it is really hurt. There is a difference between 'Wow I'm really out of shape because I haven't walked anywhere in a while' and 'My knee really hurts when I do that'. And any time you are ever in doubt seek medical attention.

Seated Activities – The body will deteriorate if it is not used. Maybe you really want to engage in physical activities but you really can't stand up for long enough to do anything meaningful. You can sit down and do many activities that are designed to get you back into the routine of regular movement. Here are a few options for you:

Marching – sit tall in your chair with your feet flat on the floor and your legs bent at a ninety-degree angle. Lift one foot and then the other, as though you are marching in the chair. Raise the knee up in the air and keep the knee bent.

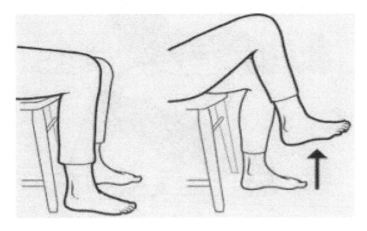

Shoulder Press – Sit tall in your chair. You can hold a set of light weights or simply make your hands into fists. If you do not own weights and do not want to buy any you can also use canned items or full water bottles. Raise your hands up into the air until your arms are straight and then lower them. Do these slowly so that your muscles will actually be doing the work.

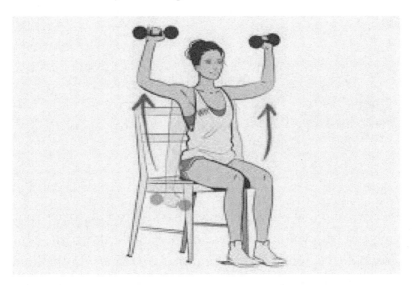

Leg lifts – This activity will strengthen your quads, which is the muscle on the front of your leg. Strong quads are needed for walking upright. Sit tall in your chair with your knees bent at ninety degrees and your feet flat on the floor. Lift a foot up into the air and away from the chair slowly; let the muscle do the work. Hold the pose for five seconds and lower it. Repeat five times on each leg.

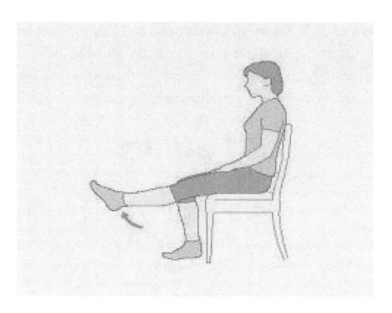

These are just a few of the activities that you can do to get yourself moving and help you in your weight loss and health goals. You are not too old to begin. You can find many routines on the internet so that you can use them alone in the privacy of your home. Remember to preview a routine before you pay for anything in case you do not like it. And many routines are offered free of charge. So do a bit of research and don't stop with one activity. Try to make your routine as varied as possible so that you will not get bored and soon you will have that body you want along with a healthier you.

Chapter Six

STAYING KETO IN REAL LIFE

Once you have spent some time at home preparing your meals and learning the ins and outs of the keto lifestyle, you might be ready to venture out in the real world again. Maybe you have lost some weight and want to debut the new you. Besides, no one really wants to stay home alone every night enjoying their own company. But can you go out in the real world and still remain on the keto diet?

The answer is yes, with a little advance planning and some strategies. Many restaurants now realize that staying relevant and remaining in business means that they will need to adapt their menus to meet the nutritional needs of various people. Simply offering a one-kind-fits-all menu will no longer work in a world where people want or need to eat a particular way and will not accept NO for an answer. And the keto diet is flexible enough that you can find menu options at any eating establishment from fast food to fine dining.

You will want to always look for fish, seafood, meat, and poultry options. Sometimes you can order just the meat portion if the daily veggie is not to your liking. If you are eating the veggie option, make sure it is one from the allowed choices and order a double portion and tell them to hold the potato. Get the salad instead of the soup and specify oil and vinegar dressing on the side. Yes, the bread and rolls will still come to the table to tempt you, but you are strong enough to resist them. If you want to order a burger or a sandwich that is fine but specify that you do not want the bread or the bun. Rice or pasta sides can be replaced by another vegetable. The vinegar and oil dressing for your salad can also be used to season your meat and vegetable options as well as butter. You can also ask for other low carb options like soy sauce, guacamole, hot sauce, vinaigrette, or béarnaise sauce.

You can still eat with friends at a fast-food restaurant. Just ask for your sandwich meat and fixings to be served in a lettuce leaf or in the container without the bun. Do not order onion rings or French fries or hash browns. Top your sandwich with mushrooms, cheese, sprouts, lettuce, bacon, and avocado. Mayonnaise is good, and ketchup is bad. Honey mustard and sweet mustard are bad, but regular yellow mustard is good. Order your chicken grilled, not fried, and have it on a salad. Stay far away from corn, baked beans, sweet potatoes, sweet and sour sauce, and barbecue sauce. A little coleslaw will be fine even though the dressing might be slightly higher in carbs than you really need.

Mexican food restaurants are great for the keto dieter. Keep your hand out of the chip basket. Just because the chips are free does not mean they are good for you. Fill your burrito with shrimp, steak, pork, or chicken and have them serve it in a bowl without the tortilla. Top your choice of meat with the onions and bell peppers used for fajitas. Extra cheese is always a good choice, both for your diet and your taste buds. Use sour cream or salsa to flavor your food. If they won't serve the burrito in a bowl (which is not likely) then just unroll it and eat the insides only. Fajitas, chili verde, carne asada, and chicken mole are all good low carb choices. Tell the server to leave the rice and beans in the kitchen and see if you can get extra sour cream, guacamole, or cheese instead.

The Asian restaurant is not the best choice for the keto dieter. Do not choose any menu item that is battered or has the word 'sweet' in its description. Order the duck without the sauce. Shirataki noodles are low carb and might be your best choice. Other good choices are green beans or sautéed cabbage or sprouts. Stir-fries and curries with low carb veggies are fine but leave the rice in the kitchen.

When you feel adventurous check out a local Indian-themed location. These restaurants are great choices for the keto dieter. Indian cuisine makes regular use of ghee (purified butter) and they put it on everything. Kebabs, curries, meat, and poultry in cream sauce, and Tandoori dishes are all great choices for you. And look for Raita on the menu. It is a creamy dip that is made from yogurt and shredded cucumbers.

One of the best options for a keto dieter is the buffet-style restaurant. You will find dozens of menu items that fit perfectly into your allowed food groups. You should eat to enjoy and don't worry about quantity. Make intentional and deliberate choices, even if it takes you a bit longer to fill up your plate. Your best places to graze will be the salad section and the meat and seafood section. There should be some good choices in the veggies also but stay away from potatoes and rice. And buffets always offer low carb condiments like oil and vinegar, sour cream, cheese, and butter. If the buffet offers sugar-free gelatin have that for dessert.

It is not impossible to follow the keto diet and have fun times with friends. Most restaurants post their menus online and many offer nutritional information. So if you know in advance where you are going you can already have your menu items picked out for when you arrive and order. Just remember that your choices are yours and do not feel the need to eat as others do. You are eating for you and that is the most important choice you will ever make.

Chapter Seven

KETO BREAKFAST RECIPES

The typical breakfast of bacon or ham and eggs is perfect on the keto diet. Just add in cheese and some type of low carb vegetable to round it out into a complete meal.

1. HUEVOS RANCHEROS

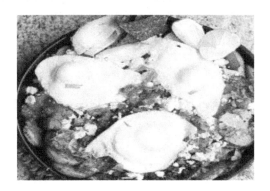

Serves one

Ingredients:

- Cilantro, fresh, one tablespoon
- Yellow onion, one half, chopped
- Avocado, one half
- Garlic, two cloves, minced
- Eggs, two,
- Tomato, one diced
- Salt, one quarter teaspoon
- Black pepper, one teaspoon
- Jalapeno, one fresh, minced
- Orange bell pepper, one half, chopped
- Coconut oil, two tablespoons

Instructions:

Fry the onion, garlic, bell pepper, and jalapeno in half of the coconut oil for five minutes. Pour in the diced tomatoes and fry for an additional five minutes. Beat the eggs in a small bowl and pour over the veggie mix in the skillet, stirring frequently until the eggs are scrambled to desired consistency. Serve with slices of fresh avocado.

Nutrition per serving:

Calories 610, 16 grams net carbs, 51 grams fat, 16 grams protein

2. ITALIAN BREAKFAST CASSEROLE

Serves four

Ingredients:

- Eggs, eight
- Butter, two tablespoons
- Cheddar cheese, five ounces shredded
- Black pepper, one teaspoon
- Salt, one half teaspoon
- Basil, fresh, chopped, one half cup
- Heavy whipping cream, one cup
- Italian sausage, fresh, twelve ounces
- Cauliflower, seven ounces

Instructions

Heat oven to 375. Use lard or oil to grease an eight by eight or nine by nine baking pan. Rinse the cauliflower well and pat it dry, and then chop the cauliflower into small bite-sized pieces. Cook the cauliflower in the melted butter for five minutes, then put it off to the side. Drop the Italian sausage into the skillet and use a firm spatula to chop it up into crumbly pieces. Fry the sausage until it is completely done and dump it into the baking pan with the cauliflower. Beat well together with the pepper, salt, heavy cream, cheddar cheese, and eggs until well mixed. Pour this mixture over the sausage and sprinkle the basil all over the top. Bake the casserole for forty minutes.

Nutrition per serving:

Calories 875, 5 grams net carbs, 79 grams fat, 34 grams protein

3. VEGETARIAN BREAKFAST CASSEROLE

Serves four

Ingredients:

- Eggs, twelve
- Black pepper, one teaspoon
- Salt, one teaspoon
- Onion powder, one teaspoon
- Leek, one half of one
- Green olives, one half cup
- Parmesan cheese, one ounce shredded
- Cherry tomatoes, one half cup
- Shredded cheese, seven ounces
- Heavy whipping cream, one cup

Instructions

Heat oven to 400. Rinse the portion of the leek and trim off the ends, then slice it very thinly. Use lard or oil to grease a thirteen by nine baking pan and lay the leeks in the bottom with the olives. Use a medium-sized bowl to beat together the onion powder, pepper, salt, eggs, cream, and the shredded cheese. Pour all of this mixture over the leeks and olives; do not worry if the leeks and olives move. Top the egg mixture with sprinkles of the parmesan cheese and the cherry tomatoes. Bake for forty minutes.

Nutrition per serving:

Calories 621, 5 grams net carbs, 52 grams fat, 33 grams protein

4. CAULIFLOWER HASH BROWNS

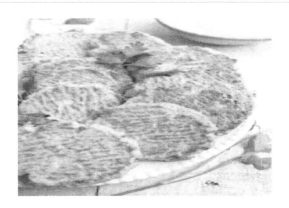

Serves four

Ingredients:

- Eggs, three well beaten
- Butter, four tablespoons
- Yellow onion, one half grated
- Black pepper, one teaspoon
- Salt, one teaspoon
- Cauliflower, one head

Instructions

Wash and rinse the cauliflower and let drain well and then pat it dry. Grate the raw cauliflower finely using a hand grater or a food processor. Dump the finely grated cauliflower into a bowl and add the salt, pepper, egg, and onion. Mix all of this together very well. Form the grated cauliflower mixture into pancake shapes and fry them in the melted butter five minutes on each side. If they do not fry long enough, they will break apart when you flip them or remove them from the pan, so do not try to rush them.

Nutrition per serving:

Calories 282, 5 grams net carbs, 26 grams fat, 7 grams protein

5. OATMEAL

Serves one

Ingredients:

- Almond milk, unsweetened, one cup
- Flaxseed, whole, one tablespoon
- Sunflower seeds, one tablespoon
- Chia seeds, one tablespoon
- Salt, one half teaspoon

Instructions

Dump all of the ingredients together into a small pan and bring the mixture to a boil in a saucepan over medium heat. When it comes to a boil, reduce the heat and allow the mix to simmer gently for two to three minutes until the mix is the desired thickness. Drop a pat of butter on the top and enjoy.

Nutrition per serving:

Calories 621, 9 grams net carbs, 62 grams fat, 10 grams protein

6. COCONUT CREAM WITH BERRIES

Serves one

Ingredients:

- Coconut cream, one half cup
- Vanilla extract, one teaspoon
- Strawberries, fresh, two ounces

Instructions

Mix the ingredients together well by using a hand mixer or an immersion mixer if one is available. An added teaspoon of coconut oil will increase the amount of fat in this dish.

Nutrition per serving:

Calories 415, 9 grams net carbs, 42 grams fat, 5 grams protein

7. SEAFOOD OMELET

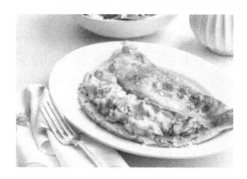

Serves two

Ingredients:

- Shrimp, cooked, five ounces
- Eggs, six
- Butter, two tablespoons
- Olive oil, two tablespoons
- Chives, fresh or dried, one tablespoon
- Mayonnaise, one half cup
- Cumin, ground, one half teaspoon
- Thyme, one quarter teaspoon
- Garlic, two cloves minced
- Red chili pepper, one diced
- Salt, one half teaspoon
- White pepper, one teaspoon

Instructions

Toss the shrimp with the olive oil until it is completely covered and fry it gently with the cumin, garlic, salt, chili pepper, and pepper for five minutes. While the shrimp mix cools beat the eggs and pours them into the skillet. Let the eggs sit undisturbed while they cook until the edges begin to brown and the center has mostly set firm. Then add the chives and the mayonnaise to the shrimp mixture. Pour the shrimp mixture onto the egg that is frying in the skillet and fold the omelet in half, frying for an additional three minutes on each side.

Nutrition per serving:

Calories 872, 4 grams net carbs, 83 grams fat, 27 grams protein

8. SPINACH AND PORK WITH FRIED EGGS

Serves two

Ingredients:

- Spinach, baby, two cups
- Pork loin, smoked, six ounces cut into chunks
- Eggs, four
- Salt, one half teaspoon
- Black pepper, one teaspoon
- Walnuts, chopped, one quarter cup
- Cranberries, one quarter cup frozen
- Butter, three tablespoons

Instructions

Wash, dry, and chop the baby spinach. Fry the spinach in the butter for five minutes stirring continuously. Remove the spinach from the pan and let it drain on a paper towel. Fry the chunks of pork loin in the same skillet for five minutes. Remove the pork from the skillet and then put the cooked baby spinach back in, adding the nuts and cranberries. Stir constantly while this is cooking for five minutes. Pour the mix into a bowl. Fry the eggs and place two on each plate with half of the spinach mixture. Serve with the chunks of fried pork loin.

Nutrition per serving:

Calories 1033, 8 grams net carbs, 99 grams fat, 26 grams protein

9. SMOKED SALMON SANDWICH

Serves two

Ingredients:

TOPPING

- Eggs, four
- Chives, fresh, chop, one tablespoon
- Smoked salmon, three ounces
- Heavy whipping cream, two tablespoons
- Salt, one half teaspoon
- White pepper, one half teaspoon
- Kale, one-ounce chop fine
- Butter, two tablespoons
- Chili powder, one quarter teaspoon
- Olive oil, two tablespoons

SPICY PUMPKIN BREAD

- Lard, one tablespoon
- Pumpkin puree, fourteen ounces
- Coconut oil, .25 cup
- Eggs, three
- Pumpkin seeds, one third cup
- Walnuts, chopped, one third cup
- Baking powder, one tablespoon
- Pumpkin pie spice, two tablespoons
- Flaxseed, one half cup
- Coconut flour, one and one quarter cups

- Almond flour, one and one quarter cups
- Psyllium husk powder, ground, two tablespoons
- Salt, one teaspoon

Instructions

Heat oven to 400. Use the lard to grease a nine by nine pan. Add the baking powder, pumpkin pie spice, nuts, psyllium husk powder, flaxseed, both flours, salt, and seeds into a bowl and mix together well. Use a separate bowl to cream together the oil, pumpkin puree, and egg. Gently pour this mixture into the dry ingredients and fold both together until all of the ingredients are well moistened. Spoon this entire mixture into the greased baking pan and bake it for one hour. Allow the bread to cool completely.

When the bread is done beat together the cream and eggs with the pepper and salt. Scramble the egg mix in the melted butter for five minutes, stirring constantly and then mix in the chili powder. Slice off two slices of the pumpkin bread and place them in the toaster to toast for three minutes. Butter the toasted pumpkin bread and lay each slice on a plate. Top each slice with the kale and the smoked salmon. Place the eggs on top of this and sprinkle with the chives.

Nutrition per serving:

Calories 678, 3 grams net carbs, 55 grams fat, 41 grams protein

10. SHRIMP DEVILED EGGS

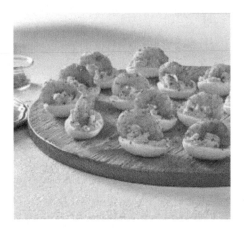

Serves four

Ingredients:

- Chives, chopped, one teaspoon
- Mayonnaise, one quarter cup
- Eggs, four, hard boiled
- Dill sprigs, eight fresh
- Tabasco sauce, one teaspoon
- Shrimp, peeled and deveined, eight large fully cooked*
- Salt, one half teaspoon
- White pepper, one half teaspoon

Instructions

Carefully peel the chilled hard-boiled eggs and then cut them in half the long way and remove the yolks. Put the yolks into a bowl and use a dinner fork to gently mash the yolks and then add the Tabasco, salt, and mayonnaise. Mix all of this together well and then carefully spoon the mixture back into the egg whites. Top each egg with one cooked shrimp and a sprig of dill.

Shrimp are sold whole or peeled and deveined. You can peel them yourself and remove the vein but the cost difference to buy them already peeled and deveined (P & D) in very small and worth the price.

Nutrition per serving:

Calories 163, .5 grams net carbs, 15 grams fat, 7 grams protein

11. SCRAMBLED EGGS WITH HALLOUMI CHEESE

Serves two

Ingredients:

- Eggs, four
- Bacon, four slices
- Salt, one half teaspoon
- Black pepper, one teaspoon
- Chili powder, one quarter teaspoon
- Black olives, pitted if needed, one half cup
- Parsley, fresh, one half cup chop fine
- Scallions, two
- Olive oil, two tablespoons
- Halloumi cheese, diced from a block, three ounces

Instructions

Chop finely the bacon and the cheese. Fry the bacon and the cheese with the scallions in the olive oil for five minutes. While this mixture is frying beat the eggs well with the parsley, pepper, chili powder, and salt. Dump the egg mix onto the bacon cheese mix in the skillet and scramble all together for three minutes while stirring constantly. Add in the olives and cook for three more minutes.

Nutrition per serving:

Calories 667, 4 grams carbs, 59 grams fat, 28 grams protein

12. COCONUT PORRIDGE

Serves one

Ingredients:

- Egg, one
- Salt, one quarter teaspoon
- Coconut oil, one tablespoon
- Coconut cream, four tablespoons
- Psyllium husk powder, ground, one half teaspoon
- Coconut flour, one tablespoon

Instructions

Pour all of the ingredients listed into a pan and mix together well. Cook this mixture over very low heat while stirring constantly until the mixture is the thickness that you desire. Serve the porridge with a spoonful of coconut milk or heavy whipping cream and a few frozen or fresh berries if you like.

Nutrition per serving:

Calories 486, 4 grams net carbs, 49 grams fat, 9 grams protein

13. WESTERN OMELET

Serves two

Ingredients:

- Eggs, six
- Smoked deli ham, five ounces diced small
- Butter, two tablespoons
- Green bell pepper, one-half cup finely chopped
- Yellow onion, one-quarter cup finely chopped
- Shredded sharp cheddar cheese, three ounces
- Sour cream, two tablespoons
- Salt, one half teaspoon
- Black pepper, one teaspoon
- Chives, chopped, one tablespoon
- Thyme, one quarter teaspoon

Instructions

Cream together the eggs and the sour cream together until they are fluffy and season this mix with salt, chives, thyme, and pepper. Sprinkle in just half of the shredded cheese and mix it together well. Cook the peppers, onion, and ham in the melted butter for five minutes while stirring often. Dump the egg mixture carefully over the ham mixture in the skillet and cook for an additional five minutes just sitting still, do not stir. Sprinkle the remainder of the shredded cheese onto the omelet and carefully fold it in half and fry for five more minutes, two and one-half minutes per side.

Nutrition per serving:

Calories 702, 6 grams net carbs, 58 grams fat, 40 grams protein

14. MUSHROOM OMELET

Serves one

Ingredients:

- Eggs, three
- Shredded cheese any style, one ounce
- Mushrooms, one half cup
- Yellow onion, diced fine, one quarter cup
- Salt, one half teaspoon
- White pepper, one quarter teaspoon
- Rosemary, one half teaspoon
- Butter, one tablespoon

Instructions

Break the eggs into a bowl carefully and season them with the pepper, salt, and rosemary. Use a fork or a hand mixer to beat the eggs until they are well mixed and slightly frothy. Pour the egg mixture into the melted butter into the pan. Let the omelet cook over medium heat until the half-inch outer edge has begun to look brown and firm and the center half is still slightly raw and wet. Sprinkle the mushrooms, onions, and cheese onto the omelet, staying mostly near the center and away from the cooked edges. Use a spatula to work the edges free of the omelet off the pan and flip one side over onto the other half. Let the omelet cook five more minutes and remove it from the pan.

Nutrition per omelet:

Calories 510, 4 grams net carbs, 43 grams fat, 25 grams protein

15. FRITTATA WITH FRESH SPINACH

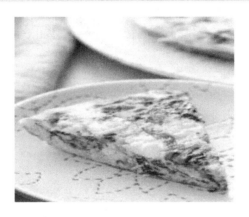

Serves four

Ingredients:

- Eggs, eight
- Heavy whipping cream, one cup
- Salt, one teaspoon
- Black pepper, one teaspoon
- Rosemary, one half teaspoon
- Thyme, one quarter teaspoon
- Shredded sharp cheddar cheese, five ounces
- Spinach, fresh, one cup washed and dried
- Butter, two tablespoons

Instructions

Heat oven to 350. Use one tablespoon of lard to grease a nine by nine-inch baking pan. Use one tablespoon of the butter to fry the bacon in a skillet over medium heat. When the bacon is crispy place the cleaned spinach in the skillet and cooks it until the spinach wilts. The bacon will break into pieces while you are stirring it with the spinach. During the time the bacon is cooking beat the eggs and the heavy cream together in a small bowl. Pour this mix into the baking pan, then add in the spinach and bacon mix and sprinkle all over the top with the sharp cheddar cheese. Bake for thirty minutes and serve hot.

Nutrition per serving:

Calories 661, 4 grams net carbs, 59 grams fat, 27 grams protein

16. CLASSIC EGGS AND BACON

Serves four

Ingredients:

- Eggs, eight
- Bacon, eight slices
- Parsley, freshly chopped, for garnish
- Cherry tomatoes, one half cup cut in half

Instructions

Fry the bacon in a skillet to desired crispiness and drain it on a paper towel. Leave at least three tablespoons of the leftover bacon grease in the skillet to use to cook the eggs any way you choose—fried or scrambled. When the eggs have almost finished cooking drop the cherry tomatoes into the skillet so that they will be slightly warmed. Serve the eggs with two strips of bacon per person and the warm cherry tomatoes on the side with fresh parsley overall for garnish and taste.

Nutrition per serving:

Calories 272, 1-gram net carbs, 22 grams fat, 15 grams protein

17. PANCAKES WITH BERRIES AND WHIP CREAM

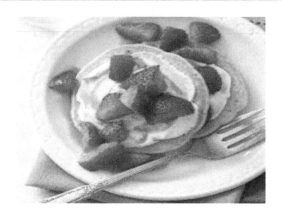

Serves four

Ingredients:

<u>TOPPING</u>

- Heavy whipping cream, one cup cold
- Berries, one cup of strawberries, raspberries, or blackberries

<u>PANCAKE</u>

- Eggs, four
- Butter, two tablespoons
- Psyllium husk powder, ground, one tablespoon
- Cottage cheese, seven ounces

Instructions

Mix the psyllium husk, cottage cheese, and the eggs together well in a small bowl. Let this mix sit for ten minutes so it will thicken. Use a large skillet to melt the butter completely over medium heat. Use a serving spoon or a ladle to pour pancake batter into the hot butter. Make the pancakes about four inches across. Fry each pancake for four minutes on each side. While the pancakes are cooking place the heavy cream in a bowl and whip with a hand mixer until the cream makes soft peaks. Place the cooked pancakes on a plate and top with the whipped cream and the berries of your choice.

Nutrition per serving:

Calories 425, 5 grams net carbs, 39 grams fat, 13 grams protein

18. MEXICAN SCRAMBLED EGGS

Serves four

Ingredients:

- Eggs, six
- Pickled jalapenos, two chopped fine
- Scallion, one chopped fine
- Butter, two tablespoons
- Shredded cheese, three ounces
- Tomato, one medium chopped fine
- Salt, one half teaspoon
- Black pepper, one teaspoon
- Chili powder, one teaspoon

Instructions

Use a medium-sized skillet over low heat to melt all of the butter and then cook the scallions, jalapenos, and tomatoes for three minutes. Beat the eggs until well mixed and pour them into the pan with the fried vegetables. Scramble the eggs to the desired degree of doneness, adding in the salt, pepper, and chili powder while you stir the eggs. When the eggs are almost done pour in the shredded cheese, stir once, and serve.

Nutrition per serving:

Calories 229, 2 grams net carbs, 18 grams fat, 14 grams protein

19. EGGS WITH AVOCADO

Serves four

Ingredients:

- Eggs, eight
- Avocado, one peeled and cut into eight slices
- Mayonnaise, full fat
- Salt and pepper to taste

Instructions

In a medium-sized pot boil four cups of water. Use a serving spoon to carefully immerse the eggs, one at a time, into the boiling water. Boil the eggs for the time that will give the result desired: eight minutes for hard-boiled, six minutes for medium eggs, and four minutes for soft boiled eggs. Serve the eggs two to a plate with a spoonful of mayonnaise on each plate and two slices of fresh avocado.

Nutrition per serving:

Calories 316, 1-gram net carbs, 29 grams fat, 11 grams protein

20. AVOCADO EGGS WITH BACON

Serves four

Ingredients:

- Eggs, hard-boiled, two
- Avocado, one half
- Salt, one half teaspoon
- Black pepper, one teaspoon
- Thyme, one quarter teaspoon
- Bacon, two ounces
- Olive oil, one teaspoon

Instructions

Heat oven to 350. Use a large spoon to place the eggs carefully into a pan of boiling water and boil them for eight minutes. Immediately place the boiled eggs into a bowl of cold water to make them easier to peel. Carefully peel the boiled eggs and then cut them in half along the length and gently remove the yolks. Put the yolks into a bowl, add the avocado and the oil and mix all these ingredients together well. Add the thyme, pepper, and salt and mix well. Fry the bacon in a skillet until it is crispy or bakes it in the heated oven while you are preparing the eggs. Spoon the egg mix carefully back into the egg white halves and top with bits of crispy crumbled bacon.

Nutrition per serving:

Calories 144, 1-gram net carbs, 13 grams fat, 5 grams protein

21. BUTTERED ASPARAGUS WITH CREAMY EGGS

Serves four

Ingredients:

- Eggs, four
- Butter, five tablespoons divided into two tablespoons and three tablespoons
- Sour cream, one half cup
- Asparagus, twenty-four ounces
- Parmesan cheese, grated, three ounces
- Lemon juice, two tablespoons
- Olive oil, one tablespoon
- Cayenne pepper, one quarter teaspoon
- Salt, one half teaspoon

Instructions

Scramble the eggs in the two tablespoons of butter until they are thoroughly cooked but still slightly wet. Pour the eggs into a blender while they are still hot and add the salt, pepper, parmesan cheese, and sour cream. Blend until this mix is smooth and creamy. Fry the asparagus in a skillet in the olive oil for five minutes. Add in the three tablespoons of butter to the skillet and let it melt completely. Turn off the heat and add in the lemon juice and let the mix set well. After ten minutes return the pan to the heat, add in the asparagus, and stir to mix completely. Place all items on a plate and serve.

Nutrition per serving:

Calories 527, 6 grams net carbs, 48 grams fat, 18 grams protein

22. NO BREAD BREAKFAST SANDWICH

Serves four

Ingredients:

- Eggs, four
- Smoked deli ham, two ounces
- Cheddar cheese, two thick slices from a block, about one-half-inch thick
- Tabasco sauce, one half teaspoon
- Salt, one half teaspoon
- Black pepper, one teaspoon
- Butter, two tablespoons

Instructions

Fry the eggs to over medium in the melted butter and then sprinkle them with salt and pepper. Place one fried egg on each of four plates for serving, one on each plate Top each egg with one slice of cheese and half of the ham. Drizzle each stack with tabasco sauce.

Nutrition per serving:

Calories 354, 2 grams net carbs, 30 grams fat, 20 grams protein

23. MUSHROOM AND CHEESE FRITTATA

Serves four

Ingredients:

<u>VINAIGRETTE</u>

- Olive oil, four tablespoons
- White wine vinegar, one tablespoon
- Black pepper, ground, one teaspoon
- Salt, one half teaspoon

<u>FRITTATA</u>

- Mushrooms, button, one cup
- Parsley, chopped from fresh, one tablespoon
- Scallions, six diced
- Kale, rinsed and dried, two cups
- Mayonnaise, one cup
- Butter, three tablespoons
- Shredded cheese, one cup
- Eggs, ten
- Black pepper, ground, one teaspoon
- Salt, one half teaspoon

Instructions

Heat oven to 350. Pour all of the vinaigrette ingredients into a jar with a lid. Shake this very well and set it aside. Fry the mushrooms, parsley, and scallions with the pepper and salt added for five minutes in the melted butter. In a different bowl mix together well the mayonnaise, cheese, and eggs. Add the scallion, mushroom, and parsley mix to the egg mix and pour all of it into a greased eight by eight-inch baking dish. Bake the frittata for forty minutes. Serve with drizzles of the vinaigrette.

Nutrition per serving:

Calories 1061, 6 grams net carbs, 101 grams fat, 32 grams protein

24. EGG MUFFINS

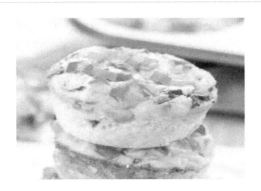

Serves six

Ingredients:

- Eggs, twelve
- Bacon, cooked, six slices
- Scallions, two, chopped finely
- Salt, one teaspoon
- Pepper, one teaspoon
- Pesto, red or green, two tablespoons
- Rosemary, one teaspoon
- Thyme, one quarter teaspoon
- Shredded cheddar cheese, one half cup
- Shredded mozzarella cheese, one half cup

Instructions

Heat oven to 350. Set paper or foil baking cups in all twelve cups of a twelve-cup muffin pan. Chop the scallions and the bacon and put a little bit in each cup. Beat the eggs with the cheese, thyme, rosemary, pesto, salt, and pepper. Divide the egg mixture into the baking cups. Bake them for twenty minutes.

Nutrition per serving:

Calories 336, 2 grams net carbs, 26 grams fat, 23 grams protein

25. CHIA PUDDING

Serves one

Ingredients:

- Cinnamon, one tablespoon
- Coconut milk, one cup
- Vanilla extract, one teaspoon
- Chia seeds, two tablespoons

Instructions

Place all of the ingredients into a glass jar or bowl. Mix together and cover well and place in the refrigerator overnight or for at least four hours. The pudding will thicken during that time, and the chia seeds will have gelled, making this a smooth, creamy breakfast pudding.

Nutrition per serving:

Calories 461, 7 grams net carbs, 44 grams fat, 7 grams protein

26. SALMON FILLED AVOCADO

Serves two

Ingredients:

- Avocados, two
- Lemon juice, two tablespoons
- Salt, one half teaspoon
- Black pepper, one teaspoon
- Sour cream, one cup
- Smoked salmon, six ounces

Instructions

Gently peel the raw avocados and cut them in half the long way and then remove the pit. Spoon the sour cream into the holes where the pit was and place the smoked salmon on top of the sour cream. Drizzle on the lemon juice and then season to taste with the salt and the pepper.

Nutrition per serving:

Calories 911, 6 grams net carbs, 71 grams fat, 58 grams protein

27. RUTABAGA FRITTERS WITH AVOCADO

Serves four

Ingredients:

MAYONNAISE DRESSING

- Ranch seasoning, one tablespoon
- Mayonnaise, one cup

FRITTERS

- Eggs, four
- Butter, for frying, four tablespoons
- Rutabaga, fifteen ounces
- Pepper, one half teaspoon
- Salt, one half teaspoon
- Halloumi cheese, eight ounces
- Turmeric, one quarter teaspoon
- Coconut flour, three tablespoons

Serve with avocado slices and leafy greens of your choice

Instructions

Heat oven to 250. Rinse the rutabaga well and peel it. Grate the rutabaga finely using a food processor or a hand grater. Use the same process for shredding the cheese. Use a large bowl to mix the coconut flour with the grated rutabaga, pepper, salt, cheese, turmeric, and eggs and let this mixture stand for ten minutes. Form the mixture into twelve equal-sized patties and fry them, three or four at a time, in the melted butter over medium heat. Fry the patties for five minutes on each side. Put the already cooked patties in the oven to keep them warm while you are cooking the rest. Top with the ranch dressing to serve.

Nutrition per serving:

Calories 1211, 14 grams net carbs, 113 grams fat, 25 grams protein

28. BACON MUSHROOM BREAKFAST CASSEROLE

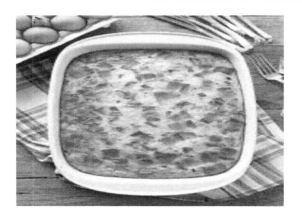

Serves four

Ingredients:

- Eggs, eight
- Bacon, twelve ounces
- Heavy whipping cream, one cup
- Butter, two tablespoons
- Salt, one teaspoon
- Pepper, one teaspoon
- Cheddar cheese, shredded, five ounces
- Mushrooms, six ounces

Instructions

Heat oven to 400. Rinse and dry the mushrooms and chop them. Chop the bacon into bite-size pieces. Fry the bacon bits and the mushrooms in the butter for five minutes over medium heat. Use one tablespoon of lard to grease a nine by thirteen-inch baking dish and add the mushroom and bacon mixture to it. Beat the cream with the eggs, cheese, pepper, and salt in a bowl and pour into the baking dish on top of the bacon and mushrooms. Bake this for forty minutes.

Nutrition per serving:

Calories 876, 6 grams net carbs, 81 grams fat, 31 grams protein

29. BAKED EGGS

Serves one

Ingredients:

- Eggs, two
- Ground pork, three ounces cooked
- Shredded cheddar cheese, two ounces

Instructions

Heat oven to 400. Use one tablespoon of lard to grease a small baking pan about a five by five-inch. Lay the cooked ground pork in the pan. Then crack both eggs and over the top of the cooked pork. Sprinkle all over the top with shredded cheese and bake for fifteen minutes.

Nutrition per serving:

Calories 509, 2 grams net carbs, 36 grams fat, 42 grams protein

30. KETO BLUEBERRY MUFFINS

Serves six to twelve

Ingredients:

- Lemon zest, one tablespoon
- Blueberries, fresh, one half cup
- Vanilla, one teaspoon
- Eggs, three large
- Almond milk, unsweetened
- Butter, one-third cup melted
- Salt, one half teaspoon
- Baking soda, one half teaspoon
- Baking powder, one and one half teaspoon
- Almond flour, two and one half cups

Instructions

Heat oven to 350. Use paper or foil liners to line all twelve cups of a twelve cup muffin pan. Use a large bowl to mix the almond flour with the salt, baking soda, and baking powder. Then mix in the vanilla, eggs, almond milk, and melted butter just until the dry ingredients are wet. Then gently fold in the lemon zest and the blueberries until they are mixed evenly into the batter. Divide the batter among the twelve cups until all of the batter is used. Bake the muffins twenty to twenty-five minutes until a knife inserted in the center of one comes out clean. Let them cool slightly before eating.

Nutrition per muffin:

Calories 229, 4 grams net carbs, 19 grams fat, 8 grams protein

31. TACO BREAKFAST SKILLET

Serves six

Ingredients:

- Cilantro, two tablespoons fresh torn
- Jalapeno, one sliced
- Salsa, one quarter cup
- Green onions, two sliced thin
- Black olives, one quarter cup sliced
- Avocado, one medium peeled, pitted, cubed
- Roma tomato, one diced
- Heavy cream, one quarter cup
- Sharp cheddar cheese, shredded, one and one-half cup divided
- Eggs, ten
- Water, two-thirds cup
- Taco seasoning, four tablespoons
- Ground beef, one pound

Instructions

Heat oven to 375. Cook the ground beef until fully cooked in a large skillet over medium heat. Drain off the excess fat. Add the taco seasoning and the water to the meat back in the skillet. Turn the heat down to low and let the mix simmer until the water has almost disappeared and the seasoning is coating the meat, for about five minutes. Beat the eggs together well in a large bowl and add the heavy cream and one cup of the cheese and mix well. Pour the meat mixture into a greased nine by nine baking dish and pour the egg mixture on top. Bake this for thirty minutes. Cover the mix with the rest of the shredded cheese, green onion, olives, tomato, and avocado. Serve with the cilantro, jalapeno, salsa, and sour cream on the side for garnish.

Nutrition per serving:

Calories 563, 9 grams carbs, 44 grams fat, 32 grams protein

32. CREAM CHEESE PANCAKES

Serves one

Ingredients:

- Cinnamon, one teaspoon
- Eggs, two
- Cream cheese, two ounces
- Butter, two tablespoons

Instructions

Make a smooth batter by mixing well all of the ingredients. Let the batter rest for five minutes. Pour in one-quarter of the batter into melted butter in a skillet over medium heat. Cook all of the pancakes for about two to three minutes on each side. Serve them with fruit if desired.

Nutrition info:

Calories 344, 3 grams net carbs, 29 grams fat, 17 grams protein

33. KETO CLOUD BREAD

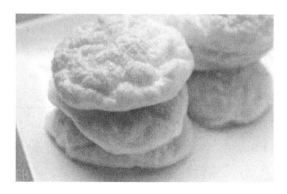

This recipe is perfect for any meal. Have it for breakfast with a bit of keto strawberry jam as an occasional treat. And look for the strawberry jam recipe in this book.

Ingredients:

- Salt, one quarter teaspoon
- Cream of tartar, one quarter teaspoon
- Cream cheese, three tablespoons at room temperature
- Eggs, three at room temperature

Instructions

Heat oven to 350. Cover two cookie sheets with parchment paper. Separate the three eggs and put the whites in one bowl and the yolks in another. Blend the cream cheese into the egg yolks. Add cream of tartar and salt to the egg whites and beat them with a hand mixer or stand mixer until they form stiff peaks. Slowly fold the yolk mixture into the egg white mixture using a spatula; mix until there are no yellow streaks remaining. Spoon the mixture onto the parchment paper covered cookie sheets in mounds about three inches across and one half inch high. Bake for thirty minutes on the middle oven rack. Allow the bread to cool completely before using.

Nutrition per piece:

Calories 35, .4 grams carbs, 2.8-gram fat, 2.2 grams protein

Chapter Eight

KETO LUNCH AND
DINNER RECIPES

These recipes will work for either lunch menus or dinner menus. A simple keto style meal for lunch or dinner would be a protein choice – meat, poultry, or fish – with a low carb vegetable choice or a leafy salad. But sometimes you want to make something creative or show off an impressive dish for a dinner party. These recipes will delight family and friends alike.

1. TUNA CASSEROLE

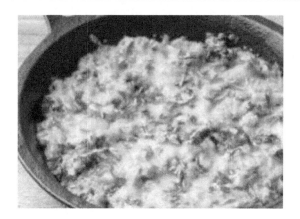

Serves four

Ingredients:

- Tuna in oil, sixteen ounces, drained
- Butter, two tablespoons
- Salt, one half teaspoon
- Black pepper, one teaspoon
- Chili powder, one teaspoon
- Celery, six stalks
- Green bell pepper, one
- Yellow onion, one
- Parmesan cheese, grated, four ounces
- Mayonnaise, one cup

Instructions

Heat the oven to 400. Chop the onion, bell pepper, and celery very fine and fry in the melted butter for five minutes. Stir together with the chili powder, parmesan cheese, tuna, and mayonnaise. Use lard

to grease an eight by eight-inch or nine by a nine-inch baking pan.
Add the tuna mixture into the fried vegetables and spoon the mix
into the baking pan. Bake it for twenty minutes.

Nutrition per serving:

Calories 953, 5 grams net carbs, 83 grams fat, 43 grams protein

2. WHITE FISH WITH CURRY AND COCONUT

Serves four

Ingredients:

- Whitefish or salmon, twenty-five ounces approximately in four pieces
- Salt, one teaspoon
- Pepper, one teaspoon
- Broccoli or cauliflower, two cups
- Cilantro, fresh, chopped, one half cup
- Coconut cream, fourteen ounces
- Curry paste, green or red, two tablespoons
- Butter or ghee, four tablespoons
- Lard to grease baking pan

Instructions

Heat the oven to 400. Use two tablespoons of lard to grease a nine by thirteen-inch baking pan and lay the fish pieces in it. Salt and pepper the fish pieces and lay a pat of butter on top of each slice. Blend the coconut cream, curry paste, and chopped cilantro in a bowl until smooth and then spoon this mix over the fish. Bake the fish for twenty minutes. While the fish is baking cut the cauliflower or the broccoli into bite-size florets and then boil them in salt water for five minutes.

Nutrition per serving:

Calories 880, 9 grams net carbs, 75 grams fat, 42 grams protein

3. CREAMY FISH CASSEROLE

Serves four

Ingredients:

- Whitefish, twenty-five ounces approximately, cut into four serving pieces
- Capers, small, two tablespoons
- Scallions, six
- Broccoli, sixteen ounces
- Butter, three tablespoons
- Dijon mustard, one tablespoon
- Heavy whipping cream, one and one quarter cups
- Parsley, dried, one tablespoon
- Black pepper, one teaspoon
- Salt, one teaspoon
- Olive oil, two tablespoons

Instructions

Heat the oven to 400. Rinse and dry the broccoli and cut it into florets leaving stems on. Use the oil to fry the broccoli for five minutes stirring occasionally. Add in the scallions and the capers. Fry for three minutes, stirring once. Use butter to grease a nine by thirteen-inch baking dish. Place the veggies in the baking dish. Lay the fish in on top of the veggies. In a small bowl mix the parsley, whipping cream, and the mustard and pour this mix on top of the vegetables and fish in the baking pan. Bake for thirty minutes. Lay six pats of butter on top in random places and let it melt before serving. Serve with a bowl of leafy greens.

Nutrition per serving:

Calories 822, 8 grams net carbs, 69 grams fat, 41 grams protein

4. SPINACH AND GOAT CHEESE PIE

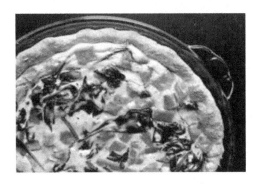

Serves six

Ingredients:

- EGG BATTER
- Sour cream, one cup
- Eggs, five
- Salt, one half teaspoon
- Black pepper, one teaspoon

<u>PIE CRUST</u>

- Almond flour, one and one half cups
- Butter, two tablespoons
- Salt, one half teaspoon
- Egg, one
- Psyllium husk powder, ground, one tablespoon
- Sesame seeds

GOAT CHEESE AND SPINACH FILLING

- Spinach, fresh, eight ounces
- Goat cheese, six ounces sliced
- Salt, one half teaspoon
- Black pepper, one teaspoon
- Cheddar cheese, shredded, one half cup
- Nutmeg, ground, one half teaspoon
- Garlic, one clove
- Butter, two tablespoons

Instructions

Heat the oven to 350. Use a fork to mix the ingredients for the dough until you make a ball of dough. Press this dough into a greased springform pan covering the bottom and the sides. Use a fork to poke holes randomly in the crust, about ten to fifteen sets. Bake the empty pie shell for ten minutes. Cream together the eggs, sour cream, salt, and pepper. Chop the garlic and the spinach fine. Fry the garlic and the spinach in the hot butter for five minutes stirring occasionally. Put this mix into the pie shell and sprinkle the grated cheese over the top. Pour the creamed egg mixture over all ingredients and place the goat cheese on top. Bake for forty-five minutes.

Nutrition per serving:

Calories 643, 4 grams net carbs, 58 grams fat, 24 grams protein

5. AVOCADO PIE

Serves four

Ingredients:

PIE CRUST

- Coconut flour, four tablespoons
- Almond flour, three-fourths of a cup
- Psyllium husk powder, ground, one tablespoon
- Sesame seeds, four tablespoons
- Water, four tablespoons
- Egg, one
- Olive oil, three tablespoons
- Salt, one quarter teaspoon
- Baking powder, one teaspoon

FILLING

- Eggs, three
- Mayonnaise, one cup
- Shredded cheese, one and one quarter cups
- Onion powder, one teaspoon
- Red chili pepper, one chop fine
- Cilantro, fresh chopped, two tablespoons
- Cream cheese, one half cup
- Salt, one half teaspoon
- Avocados, two ripe

Instructions

Heat the oven to 350. Use a fork to mix the crust ingredients in a bowl or use a food processor to mix them. Use two tablespoons of lard to grease a deep pie pan. Lay the dough ball into the pie dish, using your fingers or a spatula to spread it all over the bottom of the pan and up the sides. Poke ten to fifteen sets of holes in the bottom with a dinner fork and bake the crust empty for ten minutes. Wash and peel the avocado and remove the pit, then dice the avocado. Clean the seeds out of the chili and dice it. Mix together the diced chili and the diced avocado with the rest of the ingredients. Spoon this mix into the pre-baked crust and bake all for an additional forty minutes.

Nutrition per serving:

Calories 1146, 9 grams net carbs, 109 grams fat, 26 grams protein

6. TEX MEX STUFFED ZUCCHINI BOATS

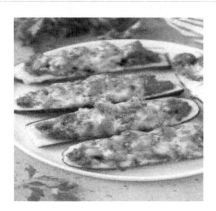

Serves four

Ingredients:

- Ground beef, one pound
- Zucchini, two medium-sized
- Cilantro, fresh, chopped fine, one half cup
- Cheddar cheese, shredded, one and one half cups
- Olive oil, one tablespoon
- Salt, one teaspoon
- Tex Mex seasoning, two tablespoons
- Olive oil or butter, two tablespoons

Instructions

Heat the oven to 400. Cut both zucchinis in half down the length and remove the seeds but do not peel. Cook the ground beef in the olive oil until it is brown, about ten minutes. Stir in the salt and the Tex Mex seasoning and let this cook until all of the liquid has cooked away. Use two tablespoons of lard to grease a nine by thirteen-inch baking pan and lay the zucchini halves in it cut side up. Stir one-third of the shredded cheese into the meat mixture and add the cilantro. Fill the halves of the zucchini evenly with the meat and cheese mix. Use the rest of the shredded cheese to sprinkle on the top. Bake the zucchini boats for twenty minutes.

Nutrition per serving:

Calories 601, 6 grams net carbs, 49 grams fat, 33 grams protein

7. BRUSSEL SPROUTS AND HAMBURGER GRATIN

Serves four

Ingredients:

- Ground beef, one pound
- Bacon, eight ounces, diced small
- Brussel sprouts, fifteen ounces, cut in half
- Salt, one teaspoon
- Black pepper, one teaspoon
- Thyme, one half teaspoon
- Cheddar cheese, shredded, one cup
- Italian seasoning, one tablespoon
- Sour cream, four tablespoons
- Butter, two tablespoons

Instructions

Heat the oven to 425. Fry bacon and Brussel sprouts in butter for five minutes. Stir in the sour cream and pour this mix into a greased eight by eight-inch baking pan. Cook the ground beef and season with the salt and pepper, then add this mix to the baking pan. Top with the herbs and the shredded cheese. Bake for twenty minutes.

Nutrition per serving:

Calories 770, 8 grams net carbs, 62 grams fat, 42 grams protein

8. ITALIAN CABBAGE STIR FRY

Serves four

Ingredients:

- Ground beef, twenty ounces
- Green cabbage, twenty-five ounces
- Tomato paste, one tablespoon
- White wine vinegar, one tablespoon
- Pepper, one teaspoon
- Salt, one teaspoon
- Onion powder, one teaspoon
- Sour cream, one cup for serving
- Basil, fresh, one half cup
- Leeks, three, slice thin
- Garlic, two cloves, chopped fine
- Rosemary, one teaspoon
- Butter, six tablespoons

Instructions

Rinse and dry the green cabbage and shred it finely. Use three tablespoons of the butter to fry the shredded cabbage for ten minutes, stirring frequently. Stir in the salt, pepper, vinegar, and onion powder and mix this well, and then remove the cabbage mix to a bowl. Place the rest of the butter into the skillet and add in the garlic and the leeks and cook these for three minutes. Pour in the meat and cook for ten more minutes, stirring often. Mix in the tomato paste and the reserved cabbage and stir well.

Nutrition per serving:

Calories 1003, 9 grams net carbs, 91 grams fat, 33 grams protein

9. TEX MEX CASSEROLE

Serves four

Ingredients:

<u>TO SERVE</u>

- Sour cream, one cup
- Scallion, one chopped fine
- Guacamole, one cup
- Leafy greens, one cup

<u>CASSEROLE</u>

- Ground beef, two pounds
- Tex Mex seasoning, three tablespoons
- Monterey Jack cheese, shredded, one cup
- Jalapenos, pickled, two ounces
- Tomatoes, crushed, seven ounces (canned is fine)
- Butter, two ounces

Instructions

Heat the oven to 400. Cook the ground beef completely in the melted butter. Add in the Tex Mex seasoning and the tomatoes and mix well. Use two tablespoons lard to grease an eight by eight-inch baking pan and put the meat mixture in it. Scatter the cheese and the jalapenos on top of the meat and bake all for twenty-five minutes. While the meat mix is baking chop up the scallion very fine and mix it with the sour cream. Serve the meat mix with a spoon of the sour cream, a spoon of guacamole, and some of the leafy greens on the side.

Nutrition per serving:

Calories 860, 8 grams net carbs, 69 grams fat, 49 grams protein

10. HERBED GRILLED CHICKEN

Serves four

Ingredients:

- Chicken thighs, eight boneless
- Dried fennel seeds, one teaspoon
- Peppercorns, whole, one teaspoon
- Garlic, minced, two teaspoons
- Thyme, dried, one tablespoon
- Rosemary, dried, one tablespoon
- Salt, one half teaspoon
- Black pepper, one teaspoon

Instructions

Mix together all of the spices with the salt and pepper in a small bowl. Press the chicken thighs into the seasoning bowl on both sides. Cover the thighs on a plate and place them in the refrigerator for two hours. Grill the thighs on a grill or cook under the broiler for eight minutes on each side. Serve with a low carb vegetable or fresh greens.

Nutrition per piece:

Calories 275, 1 gram net carbs, 17 grams fat, 1 gram protein

11. HAM CHEESE AND CHIVE SOUFFLÉ

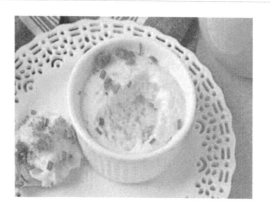

Serves four

Ingredients:

- Ham, diced, six ounces
- Cheddar cheese, shredded, one cup
- Yellow onion, one small peeled and diced
- Heavy cream, one half cup
- Eggs, six large
- Chives, chopped fresh, two tablespoons
- Salt, one teaspoon
- Black pepper, one teaspoon
- Garlic, minced, two tablespoons
- Olive oil, two tablespoons

Instructions

Heat the oven to 400. Use one tablespoon of lard to grease four six-ounce ramekins or another oven-safe dish. Fry the onion and the garlic in the olive oil for five minutes. Mix all of the remaining ingredients together in a bowl, then add the fried onions and garlic to the bowl and mix well. Divide the mix among the oven dishes and cook them for twenty-five minutes.

Nutrition per serving:

Calories 460, 5 grams net carbs, 38 grams fat, 24 grams protein

12. DEVILED EGG SALAD

Serves six

Ingredients:

- Eggs, twelve larges
- Salt, one teaspoon
- Black pepper, one teaspoon
- Green onion, two sliced thinly
- Crushed red pepper flakes, one tablespoon (optional)
- Celery, one stalk diced
- Paprika, one half teaspoon
- Apple cider vinegar
- Dijon mustard, two tablespoons
- Mayonnaise, six tablespoons

Instructions

Cook the eggs to hard-boiled by placing them in a pot of cold water, bringing the water to a boil, then boiling for ten minutes. Immediately put the pot in the sink and run cold water in it until the eggs are cooled to the touch. When the eggs have cooled completely then peel them and chop them into bite-sized chunks. In a large bowl mix together the paprika, salt, pepper, vinegar, mustard, and mayonnaise until creamy. Add in the crushed pepper (optional), celery, green onion, and the egg chunks. Keep the salad well chilled until time to serve it. Serve on a bed of leafy greens.

Nutrition per serving:

Calories 245, 1-gram net carbs, 20 grams fat, 13 grams protein

13. FAJITA CHICKEN CASSEROLE

Serves four

Ingredients:

- Chicken, fully cooked, three cups
- Yellow onion, one
- Red bell pepper, one
- Black pepper, one teaspoon
- Salt, one teaspoon
- Cheddar cheese, shredded, seven ounces or Mexican blend
- Mayonnaise, one half cup
- Cream cheese, eight ounces, softened to room temperature
- Taco seasoning, two tablespoons

Instructions

Heat the oven to 400. Peel the onion and clean the bell pepper and chop both into chunks. Keep one-third of the shredded cheese off to the side. Mix together the onion, bell pepper, mayonnaise, taco seasoning, salt, pepper, cream cheese, chicken, and the remainder of the shredded cheese. Place all of this mix into a greased eight by eight-inch or nine by nine-inch baking pan and sprinkle the reserved cheese over the top. Bake for twenty minutes.

Nutrition per serving:

Calories 1148, 10 grams net carbs, 98 grams fat, 57 grams protein

14. GARAM CHICKEN MASALA

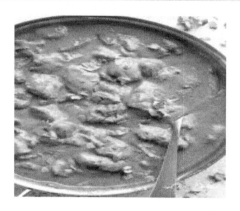

Serves four

Ingredients:

<u>CHICKEN</u>

- Chicken breast, diced into bite-size pieces, three cups

- Parsley, fresh, chopped fine, one tablespoon

- Red bell pepper, one fine diced

- Salt, one teaspoon

- Heavy whipping cream or coconut cream, one- and one-half cups

- Butter or ghee, three tablespoons

<u>GARAM MASALA</u>

- Cumin, ground, one teaspoon
- Cardamom, ground, one teaspoon

- Nutmeg, ground, one half teaspoon
- Chili powder, one teaspoon
- Ginger, ground, one teaspoon
- Turmeric, ground, one teaspoon
- Paprika, powder, one teaspoon

Instructions

Heat the oven to 400. Mix all of the Garam Masala spices together in a bowl. Fry the chicken in the melted butter over medium heat for ten minutes. Sprinkle half of the Garam Masala onto the chicken while it is cooking and mix well. Place all of the cooked chicken mixtures into a well-greased nine by thirteen-inch baking dish, including the juice in the skillet. Stir the finely diced bell pepper in with the rest of the masala mix and the coconut cream. Top the chicken in the baking dish with this mixture. Bake for thirty minutes. Sprinkle the parsley over the cooked chicken.

Nutrition per serving:

Calories 628, 6 grams net carbs, 51 grams fat, 38 grams protein

15. CHICKEN CABBAGE AND ONIONS

Serves two

Ingredients:

- Rotisserie chicken or cooked chicken breast, two cups
- Red onion, one half of medium onion
- Green cabbage, one cup finely shredded
- Pepper, one teaspoon
- Salt, one teaspoon
- Greek yogurt, one half cup
- Olive oil, one tablespoon

Instructions

Lay rounds of the shredded cabbage on two dinner plates and top these with thin slices of the red onions. Pour the olive oil over the onions and cabbage in thin lines and season with the salt and pepper. Place spoons of Greek yogurt besides the vegetable mix and top the onions and cabbage with the diced cooked chicken.

Nutrition per serving:

Calories 1041, 7 grams net carbs, 91 grams fat, 48 grams protein

16. CHICKEN LEGS WITH COLESLAW

Serves four

Ingredients:

CHICKEN

- Chicken legs, two pounds
- Olive oil, two tablespoons
- Sour cream, one half cup
- Coconut, shredded, unsweetened, three ounces
- Pork rinds, six ounces
- Olive oil, four tablespoons
- Salt, one teaspoon
- Jerk seasoning, two tablespoons

COLESLAW

- Mayonnaise, one cup
- Pepper, one teaspoon
- Salt, one half teaspoon
- Green cabbage, two cups chopped finely

Instructions

Heat the oven to 350. Mix in a bowl the sour cream with the salt and the jerk seasoning. Pour this over the chicken legs in a bowl and let them marinate for thirty minutes. Throw away the marinade. Crush the pork rinds and mix in the coconut. Roll the chicken legs in the coconut pork rind mixture. Lay the chicken legs on an oven rack that is over a baking dish or cookie sheet. Bake the chicken for forty-five minutes, turning it over after twenty minutes. During the time that the chicken is baking, you can make the coleslaw by coarsely shredding or chopping the cabbage and mixing it well with the rest of the ingredients. Serve the chicken with the slaw.

Nutrition per serving:

Calories 1370, 7 grams net carbs, 116 grams fat, 68 grams protein

17. RUTABAGA AND PAPRIKA CHICKEN

Serves four

Ingredients:

- Chicken thighs, eight boneless
- Rutabaga, one large
- Salt, one teaspoon
- Pepper one teaspoon
- Mayonnaise, one cup
- Paprika, one tablespoon
- Olive oil, four tablespoons

Instructions

Heat the oven to 400. Use two tablespoons of lard to grease a nine by thirteen-inch baking dish and lay the chicken pieces in it. Wash and dry the outside of the rutabaga and then peel it and cut it into two-inch long pieces. Add the rutabaga to the chicken in the baking dish and season both ingredients with the salt, pepper, and paprika. Pour the olive oil over the top of all the ingredients and bake for forty-five minutes uncovered. Serve with the mayonnaise on the side.

Nutrition per serving:

Calories 1165, 15 grams net carbs, 103 grams fat, 40 grams protein

18. CHICKEN BACON RANCH CASSEROLE

Serves eight

Ingredients:

- Chicken thighs, cooked and diced, two pounds
- Bacon, cooked, four slices
- Cheddar cheese, two cups shredded and divided
- Yellow onion, diced, one quarter cup
- Sour cream, one half cup
- Mayonnaise, one cup
- Cream cheese, eight ounces room temperature
- Broccoli, one pound chopped small and steamed
- Garlic powder, two teaspoons
- Parsley, chopped, one tablespoon
- Salt, one teaspoon
- Black pepper, one teaspoon

Instructions

Heat the oven to 350. Use two tablespoons of lard to grease a thirteen by nine-inch baking dish. Cream together the sour cream, mayonnaise, and cream cheese and stir in the pepper, salt, garlic powder, and parsley. Mix in the broccoli, onion, chicken, bacon, and one and one-half cups of the cheese. Put this mix into the baking pan and sprinkle the rest of the cheese over the top of the casserole and bake for thirty minutes.

Nutrition per serving:

Calories 545, 5 grams net carbs, 42 grams fat, 38 grams protein

19. PIMIENTO CHEESE MEATBALLS

Serves four

Ingredients:

MEATBALLS

- Ground beef, two pounds
- Salt, one teaspoon
- Pepper, one teaspoon
- Butter, two tablespoons for frying
- Egg, one

PIMIENTO CHEESE

- Pimientos, one quarter cup
- Mayonnaise, one half cup
- Cheddar cheese, grated, one half cup
- Cayenne pepper, one quarter teaspoon
- Dijon mustard, one tablespoon
- Paprika powder or chili powder, one teaspoon

Instructions

Put all of the ingredients for the pimiento cheese in a bowl and mix it together and let this mix sit for five minutes. Then add in the salt, pepper, egg, and ground beef and mix well with your hands or a spoon. Form the mix into golf ball-sized meatballs and fry the meatballs in the melted butter for ten minutes on each side. Serve with a salad of leafy greens on the side.

Nutrition per serving:

Calories 660, 1 gram net carbs, 53 grams fat, 42 grams protein

20. SLOPPY JOES

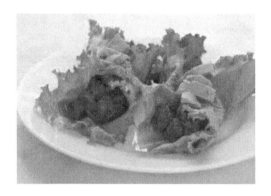

Serves four

Ingredients:

- Ground beef, one pound
- Salt, one teaspoon
- Black pepper, one teaspoon
- Worcestershire sauce, two teaspoons
- Tomato paste, one quarter cup
- Beef broth, three quarters cup
- Garlic, minced, two tablespoons
- Yellow onion, one small diced finely
- Celery, one stalk diced finely

Instructions

Cook the beef in a skillet over medium heat until it is well browned using a spatula or a spoon to break it up into small fine pieces. When the meat is thoroughly browned add in the garlic, onion, and celery and cook for five more minutes. Blend in the leftover ingredients and mix together well. Turn down the heat and let the mix simmer for twenty minutes until it begins to thicken. Serve the sloppy joes on keto cloud bread or on leaf lettuce.

Nutrition per serving:

Calories 240, 4.5 grams net carbs, 7.5 grams fat, 36 grams protein

21. PIGS IN A BLANKET

Serves six

Ingredients:

- Hot dogs, all-beef, twelve
- Mozzarella cheese, shredded, two cups
- Sesame seeds, one teaspoon
- Eggs, two whisked
- Coconut flour, one half cup
- Cream cheese, two ounces at room temperature
- Baking powder, one half teaspoon
- Oregano, dried, one teaspoon
- Garlic powder, one half teaspoon
- Onion powder, one teaspoon

Instructions

Heat oven to 400. Lay parchment paper on a cookie sheet. Put the cream cheese and mozzarella in a heatproof bowl and microwave for three minutes, then mix it together well until creamy. In another bowl mix together the eggs, baking powder, garlic powder, onion powder, oregano, and coconut flour until they are well mixed. Mix in the melted cheese. Wet your hands before sticking them in the dough because it will be sticky. Separate the dough into twelve equal-sized pieces and roll them into balls. Roll the balls of dough out into circles the same width as the hot dog is long. Roll up each hotdog with a circle of dough and lay them on the parchment paper on the cookie sheet. Sprinkle the sesame seeds on the dough and then bake for fifteen to twenty minutes until they are browned.

Nutrition per two hot dogs:

Calories 370, 7.5 grams net carbs, 23.5 grams fat, 24.5 grams protein

22. BAKED FISH STICKS

Serves four

Ingredients:

- Cod fillets, fresh, twelve ounces
- Egg, one large
- Pork rinds, one three and one half ounce bag
- Coconut flour, one and one half tablespoons

Instructions

Heat the oven to 400. Cut the codfish into strips and season them with the salt and pepper. Evenly coat the fish strips with the coconut flour. Smash the pork rinds into fine crumbs. Beat the water and egg white together well and use it to dip the fish strips into, and then into the pork rinds. Gently lay the fish sticks on a well-greased cookie sheet and bake them for fifteen minutes.

Nutrition per serving:

Calories 270, 1 gram net carbs, 11.5 grams fat, 38 grams protein

23. LEMON PARMESAN BAKED COD

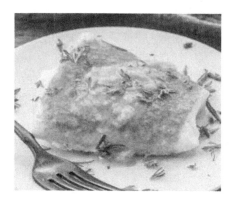

Serves four

Ingredients:

- Cod fillets, boneless, two pounds
- Lemon zest, one tablespoon
- Parsley, chopped, one tablespoon
- Paprika, one teaspoon
- Parmesan cheese, grated, three-fourths cup
- Garlic, minced, two tablespoons
- Butter, melted, one quarter cup

Instructions

Heat the oven to 400. Lay parchment paper over a cookie sheet. Cream together the garlic and butter in one bowl and mix the paprika with the parmesan in another bowl. Dip the fillets in the butter on both sides one by one and then roll them in the parmesan mixture. Lay the fillets on the cookie sheet. When all of the fillets are on the cookie sheet sprinkle them with the lemon zest and the parsley and bake for twenty minutes until the flesh of the fish separates easily with a fork.

Nutrition per serving:

Calories 320, 1 gram net carbs, 17.5 grams fat, 36.5 grams protein

24. BACON-WRAPPED MEATLOAF

Serves four

Ingredients:

- Ground beef, two pounds
- Egg, one
- Cheddar cheese, shredded, one half cup
- Heavy cream, for the gravy
- Bacon, seven slices
- Soy sauce, one tablespoon
- Black pepper, one teaspoon
- Salt, one teaspoon
- Basil, dried one teaspoon
- Oregano, dried, one teaspoon
- Mayonnaise, one half cup
- Yellow onion, one, chopped fine
- Butter, two tablespoons

Instructions

Heat the oven to 400. In the melted butter fry the onion for five minutes. Put the meat into a large bowl. Mix in the butter and onion mixture along with the remainder of the ingredients except for the bacon and the heavy cream. Use your hands to mix this together well, but do not overwork the mixture because this will make the meatloaf too dry. Use two tablespoons of lard to grease a nine-inch loaf dish. Make the meat mixture into a loaf shape and wrap the bacon around it. Bake for one hour. Remove the meat from the baking pan and pour the juices into a bowl with the whipping cream and mix well. Top the individual slices with the cream gravy mixture.

Nutrition per serving:

Calories 1038, 6 grams net carbs, 90 grams fat, 48 grams protein

25. ASIAN MEATBALLS WITH BASIL SAUCE

Serves four

Ingredients:

ASIAN MEATBALLS

- Ground pork, two pounds
- Black pepper, one teaspoon
- Ginger, ground, one tablespoon
- Coconut oil, two tablespoons
- Green cabbage, two cups shredded
- Butter, two tablespoons
- Yellow onion, minced, one half cup

BASIL SAUCE

- Mayonnaise, three-fourths cup
- Salt, one half teaspoon
- Black pepper, one half teaspoon
- Basil, fine chop, one tablespoon
- Radishes, one half cup sliced paper-thin

PICKLED ONION SALAD

- Rice vinegar, one tablespoon
- Scallions, one ounce
- Red chili pepper, one
- Salt, one half teaspoon

- Water, two tablespoons

Instructions

MEATBALLS: Heat oven to 200. Mix well all of the ingredients for the meatballs using a large spoon or your hands. Shape this mix into twenty little meatballs. Fry the meatballs in hot coconut oil for ten minutes. Put the meatballs in the oven to keep them warm. Fry the green cabbage in the melted butter over medium heat in a large skillet for ten minutes, stirring it occasionally. Arrange the cabbage on a plate and lay the meatballs on top of the cabbage. Serve the onion salad and the basil sauce on the side.

PICKLED ONION SALAD: Slice the chili pepper and the scallions thinly and mix them with the rice vinegar, water, and salt and set this mix to the side.

BASIL SAUCE: Mix the sliced radishes with the basil and the mayonnaise. Add in the salt and the pepper, mix well and set this to the side.

Nutrition per serving:

Calories 860, 9 grams net carbs, 77 grams fat, 30 grams protein

26. BACON BURGER CASSEROLE

Serves four

Ingredients:

- Ground beef, one pound
- Bacon, eight slices
- Tomatoes, two
- Dill pickles, two chopped fine
- Butter, one tablespoon
- Black pepper, one teaspoon
- Salt, one teaspoon
- Cheddar cheese, shredded, one cup
- Heavy cream, one cup
- Tomato paste, two tablespoons
- Eggs, two
- Garlic, minced, one tablespoon

Instructions

Heat the oven to 400. Fry the bacon in one tablespoon of butter for five minutes and chop into small pieces. Dump the chopped bacon back in the skillet and add in the ground beef and fry for an additional ten minutes until the beef is browned. Stir in two-thirds of the shredded cheese along with the tomatoes, the minced garlic, the seasonings, and the diced dill pickle. Use two tablespoons of lard to grease an eight by eight-inch baking pan. Mix the tomato paste, eggs, and cream in a small bowl and stir this into the meat mixture in the skillet. Put all of this mix into the baking pan and top it with the remainder of the shredded cheese. Bake for twenty minutes.

Nutrition per serving:

Calories 1041, 8 grams net carbs, 91 grams fat, 46 grams protein

27. SALMON WITH SPINACH AND PESTO

Serves four

Ingredients:

- Salmon, two pounds
- Parmesan cheese, grated, two ounces
- Pesto, green or red, one tablespoon
- Butter, one tablespoon
- Spinach, fresh, one pound
- Black pepper, one teaspoon
- Salt, one half teaspoon
- Sour cream, one cup

Instructions

Heat the oven to 400. Use two tablespoons of lard to grease a nine by a thirteen-inch baking pan. Season the salmon pieces with the salt and pepper and lay it in the baking pan with the skin down. Blend the sour cream, pesto, and parmesan cheese in a small bowl and use this mixture to coat the salmon. Bake the fish for twenty minutes. While the salmon is baking fry the spinach in the butter until it wilts, about two to three minutes. Serve the spinach with the baked salmon.

Nutrition per serving:

Calories 902, 3 grams net carbs, 78 grams fat, 45 grams protein

28. PEPPERONI PIZZA

Serves four

Ingredients:

- Pepperoni, sliced, four ounces
- Mozzarella, shredded, one and one half cups
- Tomato sauce, one cup
- Salt, one half teaspoon
- Cream of tartar, one quarter teaspoon
- Garlic powder, one teaspoon
- Whey protein powder, plain, one cup
- Eggs, three large beaten
- Water, one tablespoon
- Heavy cream, two tablespoons
- Butter, one quarter cup melted
- Cream cheese, eight ounces at room temperature

Instructions

Heat the oven to 350. Use two tablespoons of lard to grease a twelve-inch cast-iron skillet. Cream together the eggs, water, heavy cream, butter, and cream cheese. Add in the cream of tartar, salt, garlic powder, baking powder, and the protein powder. Blend all of this until it is smooth and then put it in the skillet and spread it to cover the bottom. Bake this for twenty minutes. Cover the crust with the tomato sauce, then top with the shredded cheese and add the pepperoni. Put the skillet of pizza back in the oven and bake for another ten minutes. Let the pizza cool for five minutes before cutting it.

144

Nutrition per serving:

Calories 300, 2.5 grams net carbs, 27.5 grams fat, 18.5 grams protein

29. AVOCADO SHRIMP SALAD

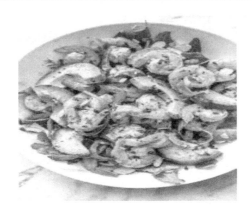

Serves four

Ingredients:

- Shrimp, one pound small size cooked, peeled, and deveined
- Cilantro, chopped fresh, two tablespoons
- Red onion, diced, one quarter cup
- Tomato, one small diced small
- Avocado, one peeled, pitted and diced
- Salt, one teaspoon
- Black pepper, one teaspoon
- Olive oil, one teaspoon
- Lime juice, one quarter cup

Instructions

Mix well the olive oil, lime juice, salt, and pepper in a medium-size bowl. Mix in the cilantro, red onion, tomato, avocado, and shrimp and mix it together well. This salad needs to be kept chilled until you are ready to serve it.

Nutrition per serving:

Calories 255, 4 grams net carbs, 13 grams fat, 27 grams protein

30. PHILLY CHEESE STEAK

Serves four

Ingredients:

- Sirloin steak, one pound
- Provolone cheese, four slices
- Sweet onion, one small sliced paper-thin
- Green pepper, one medium cleaned and sliced thin
- Salt, one teaspoon
- Black pepper, one teaspoon
- Olive oil, one tablespoon
- Keto bread, four slices

Instructions

Salt and pepper the steak and slice it into very thin strips, about one-eighth of an inch thick. Fry the steak strips in the olive oil over medium heat and cook until they are browned, five to ten minutes. Take the steak from the skillet and add in the green peppers and the onion and fry for five minutes. Lay a slice of cheese on a slice of keto bread and top with the steak slices and the onion and green pepper mixture.

Nutrition per serving:

Calories 350, 2.5 grams net carbs, 18 grams fat, 42 grams protein

Chapter Nine

SNACKS AND APPETIZERS

While the keto lifestyle does not encourage snacking between meals, there are times when you want a little something to hold you until the next meal. Or you might not be hungry enough for a full meal and a little snack will do just fine. And everyone would love to impress their guests or coworkers with a fabulous tray of goodies that they can also enjoy guilt-free. These snacks and appetizers will fit any of those situations.

1. BACON-WRAPPED SCALLOPS

Serves four

Ingredients:

- Salt, one half teaspoon
- Black pepper, one half teaspoon
- Olive oil, two tablespoons
- Bacon, eight slices cut in half, middle of the slice
- Sea scallops, sixteen
- Toothpicks, sixteen

Instructions

Heat the oven to 425. Lay parchment paper on a cookie sheet. Remove any side muscles the scallops might have and dry them with a paper towel. Use one half of a slice of bacon to wrap each scallop around and then hold the bacon to the scallop with a toothpick. Brush on the olive oil and then season with the salt and pepper. Lay the scallops on the parchment paper and bake for fifteen minutes.

Nutrition per serving:

Calories 224, 2 grams net carbs, 17 grams fat, 12 grams protein

2. BUFFALO CHICKEN JALAPENO POPPERS

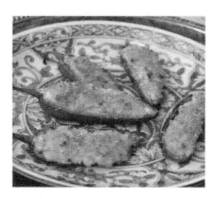

Serves five

Ingredients:

- Bacon, four slices cooked, drained, and crumbled
- Buffalo wing sauce, one quarter cup
- Mozzarella cheese, shredded, one quarter cup
- Blue cheese, crumbled, one half cup divided
- Cream cheese, four ounces at room temperature
- Salt, one half teaspoon
- Onion powder, one half teaspoon
- Garlic, minced, two tablespoons
- Chicken, ground, eight ounces
- Jalapeno peppers, ten large sizes, cut in half longways and seeds removed
- Ranch dressing and sliced green onions for serving

Instructions

Heat the oven to 350. Lay foil or parchment paper on a cookie sheet. Lay the jalapeno pepper halves on the foil or parchment paper. Cook together over medium heat the garlic, ground chicken, onion powder, and salt for about ten minutes until the chicken is fully cooked. Dump this mixture into a large bowl and mix in the wing sauce, mozzarella cheese, and one-quarter cup of the crumbled blue cheese. Put some of this mix into all of the pepper halves and top them with the bacon crumbles and the rest of the blue cheese. Bake the poppers for thirty minutes and serve with the ranch dressing and the green onions.

Nutrition for four poppers:

Calories 252, 4.6 grams net carbs, 19 grams fat, 16 grams protein

3. RUTABAGA FRIES

Serves eight

Ingredients:

- Rutabagas, two medium-sized about twenty-four ounces each
- Black pepper, one half teaspoon
- Salt, one teaspoon
- Olive oil, one quarter cup

Instructions

Heat the oven to 400. Wash and peel the rutabagas and slice them into one-quarter-inch thick circles. Slice each circle into sticks that are a one-quarter inch wide. Mix in a large bowl the sticks of rutabaga with the black pepper, salt, and olive oil. Arrange the fries on a metal rack that is sitting on top of a cookie sheet and back them for forty-five minutes.

Nutrition info per ten fries:

Calories 96, 6 grams net carbs, 6 grams fat, 1-gram protein

4. SPICY DEVILED EGGS

Makes twenty-four egg halves

Ingredients:

- Chives, minced, one teaspoon
- Chili powder, one teaspoon
- Salt, one teaspoon
- Black pepper, one teaspoon
- Dijon mustard, one tablespoon
- Sriracha sauce, one tablespoon
- Mayonnaise, one third cup
- Eggs, twelve larges

Instructions

Hard boil the eggs and when they are cool, peel them and cut them in half the long way. Remove the yolks gently and place them into a large bowl. Mash the yolks into a paste with a fork or a potato masher. Stir in the mustard, sriracha sauce, salt, pepper, chili powder, and the mayonnaise until the mix is smooth and creamy. Refill the egg whites with this mixture using a spoon or a frosting bag to pipe the mix in. When you are ready to serve the eggs top them with the chives.

Nutrition per egg half:

Calories 53, 1-gram net carbs, 4 grams fat, 2 grams protein

5. PESTO BACON AND CAPRESE SALAD SKEWERS

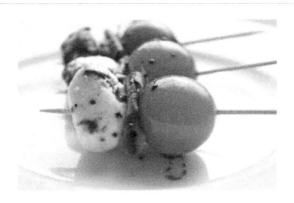

Serves 10, three skewers each

Ingredients:

- Black pepper, one teaspoon
- Salt, one teaspoon
- Olive oil, two tablespoons
- Basil pesto, one quarter cup
- Mozzarella balls or chunks, thirty pieces equaling ten ounces
- Basil, fresh, thirty leaves
- Bacon, five slices cooked and cut into six pieces each
- Grape tomatoes, thirty
- Toothpicks

Instructions

Place the food on the toothpicks in this order: mozzarella balls, basil leaf, bacon piece, and grape tomato. Mix together in a small bowl the olive oil and the pesto and drizzle it over the skewers and then sprinkle them with salt and pepper.

Nutrition info per three skewers:

Calories 153, 2 grams net carbs, 12 grams fat, 7 grams protein

6. BAKED COCONUT SHRIMP

Serves four

Ingredients:

- Black pepper, one half teaspoon
- Salt, one half teaspoon
- Paprika, one quarter teaspoon
- Garlic powder, one quarter teaspoon
- Coconut flakes, unsweetened, two cups
- Eggs, three large well beat
- Coconut flour, three tablespoons
- Medium shrimp, one pound, forty-two to forty-eight peeled and deveined, thawed

Instruction

Heat the oven to 400. Lay a wire rack onto a cookie sheet and spray it with oil spray. Set three bowls on the counter. In the first one put the beaten eggs, in the next one put the coconut flakes, and in the last one put a mix of the pepper, salt, paprika, garlic powder, and coconut flour. Dip each shrimp into the flour mixture first, then into the egg wash and then roll in the flakes of coconut. Lay them on the wire rack and bake for ten minutes, turning them over after five minutes.

Nutrition info:

Calories 443, 5 grams net carbs, 30 grams fat, 31 grams protein

7. BAKED GARLIC PARMESAN WINGS

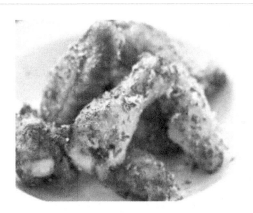

Serves six

Ingredients:

- Black pepper, one half teaspoons
- Salt, one teaspoon
- Onion powder, one teaspoon
- Garlic powder, two teaspoon
- Parsley, chopped, one tablespoon
- Garlic, minced, one tablespoon
- Parmesan cheese, grated, one half cup
- Butter, melted, one half cup
- Baking powder, two tablespoons
- Chicken wings, two pounds thawed

Instructions

Heat the oven to 250. Salt and pepper the wings and let them sit for ten minutes. Shake the baking powder over the wings and toss them so that the baking powder covers all of the wings. Spread the wings on an oven rack and bake them for thirty minutes. Change the temperature of the oven to 425 and bake the wings for another thirty minutes. Prepare the sauce for the wings while the wings are baking by mixing the onion powder, garlic powder, parsley, minced garlic, parmesan cheese, and melted butter in a bowl. When the wings have finished cooking, let them sit for five minutes and then toss them in the sauce.

Nutrition info:

Calories 468, 2 grams carbs, 38 grams fat, 30 grams protein

8. COLD CRAB DIP

Serves twelve

Ingredients:

- Chives, chopped, two tablespoons
- Crabmeat, eight ounces, press between paper towels to remove any moisture
- Old Bay seasoning, one quarter to one half teaspoon (to taste)
- Lemon juice, one teaspoon
- Sour cream, three tablespoons
- Cream cheese, four ounces at room temperature

Instructions

Cream together the lemon juice, seasoning, sour cream, and cream cheese until smooth and creamy. Gently fold in the chives and the crab meat just until mixed with the cream cheese mixture. Serve with slices of bell pepper, cucumber, or celery.

Nutrition info:

Calories 41, 0 grams net carbs, 2 grams fat, 3 grams protein

9. CHICKEN NUGGETS

Serves four

Ingredients:

- Butter, four tablespoons
- Black pepper, one half teaspoon
- Salt, one teaspoon
- Garlic powder, one teaspoon
- Onion powder, one teaspoon
- Paprika, one teaspoon
- Tapioca flour, one tablespoon
- Coconut flour, three tablespoons
- Chicken breast or tenders, one pound skinless and boneless cut into chunks

Instructions

Heat the oven to 425. Mix together in a large bowl the tapioca flour, coconut flour, salt, pepper, onion garlic, and paprika. Melt the butter and put it into a shallow pan. Coat the chicken pieces with the melted butter and then roll them in the flour mixture. Bake the nuggets for fifteen minutes, turning after eight minutes.

Nutrition info:

Calories 252, 4.2 grams net carbs, 13 grams fat, 27 grams protein

10. ONION RINGS

Serves two

Ingredients:

- Parmesan cheese, grated, one half cup
- Pork rinds, crushed, one half cup
- Heavy whipping cream, one tablespoon
- Eggs, two large
- Coconut flour, one half cup
- Onion, one white medium-sized

Instructions

Heat the oven to 425. Slice the onion into one half-inch thick rings after peeling it. You will need three different bowls for the dipping of the onion rings. Place the coconut flour in the first bowl, the mixed whipping cream and beaten egg in the second bowl, and the mixed pork rinds and parmesan cheese in the last bowl. Dip the onion rings in the flour, then the egg wash, and then the pork rind mix. Bake the onion ring in the oven for fifteen minutes.

Nutrition info:

Calories 211, 4.5 grams net carbs, 12.5 grams fat, 16 grams fat

11. SAUSAGE STUFFED MUSHROOMS

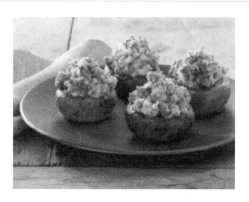

Makes twenty mushrooms

Ingredients:

- Sausage, two links any type
- Baby Bella Mushrooms, twenty
- Cheddar Cheese, one cup
- Onion, diced, one quarter cup
- Garlic, minced, two teaspoons
- Black pepper, one half teaspoon
- Salt, one half teaspoon
- Butter, two tablespoons

Instructions

Heat the oven to 350. Wash and dry the mushrooms. Pull the stalks off and chop the stalks up finely. Mix the diced stalks with the diced onions. Pull off the casing from the sausage and throw it away. Cook the sausage meat in the two tablespoons of butter in a skillet over medium heat. When the sausage is fully cooked, take it from the pan and set it aside. Put the garlic, mushroom stalks, and diced onion into the pan with the leftover liquid and cook for five minutes, stirring often. Pour this mix into a bowl and add the salt, pepper, cheddar cheese, and sausage. Fill all of the mushroom caps with the sausage mixture. Set the caps on a cookie sheet and bake the mushrooms for twenty minutes.

Nutrition info per mushroom:

Calories 56, 1.3 grams net carbs, 3.7 grams fat, 3.3 grams protein

12. PARMESAN CRISPS

Serves two

Ingredients:

- Jalapeno, one medium (optional)
- Provolone cheese, two slices
- Parmesan cheese, grated, eight tablespoons

Instructions

Heat the oven to 425. Lay parchment paper on a cookie sheet. Lay eight mounds of parmesan, one tablespoon each, on the parchment paper. If you are using the jalapeno clean out the seeds and slice the pepper as thin or as thick as you want to. Lay these slices on the parmesan cheese. Cut the slices of mozzarella into four equal squares and lay one square over the parmesan cheese and the jalapeno if you are using it. Bake these for nine minutes and allow to cool slightly before eating. These are great served with ranch dressing or sour cream.

Nutrition info per crisp:

Calories 162, 1.5 grams carbs, 10 grams fat, 14 grams protein

13. ZUCCHINI PIZZA BITES

Serves six

Ingredients:

- Pepperoni, one quarter cup mini slices

- Mozzarella cheese, one cup

- Provolone cheese, grated, one half cup

- Black pepper, one quarter teaspoon

- Salt, one half teaspoon

- Italian seasoning, one teaspoon

- Egg, one

- Zucchini, shredded, two cups

Instructions

Heat the oven to 400. Use olive oil cooking spray to spray a mini muffin pan. Lay the shredded zucchini in paper towels and squeeze out as much liquid as possible. Dump the shredded zucchini into a bowl and add the provolone cheese, salt, pepper, Italian seasoning, and egg, mixing thoroughly. Divide the mixture into the muffin cups, packing the mix down into each cup. Sprinkle the mozzarella cheese onto the cups and then top the cheese with the mini pepperonis. Bake them for fifteen to eighteen minutes. Let them sit for ten minutes before serving, using a butter knife to loosen them from the pan.

Nutrition per serving:

Calories 230, 3 grams net carbs, 9.3 grams fat, 16.4 grams fat

14. TUNA IN CUCUMBER CUPS

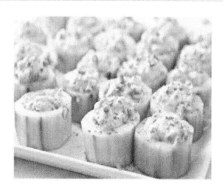

Makes ten

Ingredients:

- Dill, fresh for garnish
- Black pepper, one teaspoon
- Mayonnaise, one third cup
- Tuna, one six-ounce can
- Cucumber, one large cut into one-inch thick slices

Instructions

Use a small spoon or a melon baller to scoop most of the middle out of the slices of cucumber, leaving just a thin line at the bottom to make the cup. Put the cucumber you removed into a paper towel and press it to remove excess liquid. Chop the cucumber finely and put it into a bowl with the drained tuna, mayonnaise, and pepper. Mix this well and use a small spoon to fill the cucumber cups. Garnish with a sprig of fresh dill and serve.

Nutrition info per cup:

Calories 22, 2 grams net carbs, .7 grams fat, 2 grams protein

15. ITALIAN SUB ROLL-UPS

Serves four

Ingredients:

- Italian seasoning
- Apple cider vinegar
- Olive oil
- Lettuce, shredded
- Mayonnaise
- Provolone cheese, four slices
- Pepperoni, four slices
- Sopressata, four slices
- Mortadella, four slices
- Genoa salami, four slices
- Toothpicks

Instructions

Layout the largest slices of meat first. Then add the next smallest slices, going until all of the meat is in four stacks. Spread mayonnaise thinly on the meat, staying near the center, so it does not ooze out when you roll it up. Lay the slices of provolone cheese on the stacks. Add in some of the shredded lettuce and season with the Italian seasoning. Roll up the stacks and hold with a toothpick. Drizzle the rolls with the apple cider vinegar and the olive oil.

Nutrition info per roll:

Calories 235, 1 gram net carbs, 20 grams fat, 10 grams protein

Chapter Ten

SAUCES AND DRESSINGS

Many sauces and dressings can be store-bought but they might also have added sugars, and they will certainly have added preservatives that you may be trying to eliminate from your diet. Any sauce or dressing can be easily made at home with fresh ingredients.

1. LOW CARB STRAWBERRY JAM

Ingredients:

- Knox gelatin powder, three-fourths teaspoon
- Lemon juice, one tablespoon
- Water, one quarter cup
- Sugar replacement, one quarter cup
- Strawberries, diced, one cup

Instructions

Sprinkle the lemon juice with the gelatin and allow it to sit and thicken. Add the water, strawberries, and sugar replacement to a small pot and set it over medium heat. As soon as this mixture begins to simmer then lower the heat and let it simmer for twenty minutes. Chop up the gelatin lemon juice mix and mix it in with the warm strawberries and let it dissolve. Let the jam cool after removing the pan from the heat, then spoon the mix into a clean glass jar. This jam will remain good in the refrigerator for two weeks.

This can be made with any low carb fruit.

Nutrition info per tablespoon:

Calories 57, .85 grams net carbs, o grams fat, .66 grams protein

2. PLAIN MAYONNAISE

Ingredients:

- Lemon juice, two teaspoons
- Olive oil, one cup
- Dijon mustard, one tablespoon at room temperature
- Egg yolk, one at room temperature

Instructions

Cream together the mustard and the egg yolk and then pour in the oil slowly while stirring to mix. Add in the lemon juice and mix one last time and then let the mixture sit until it is thick. This will keep for about four days in the refrigerator.

Nutrition info per one quarter cup:

Calories 511, 0 grams net carbs, 57 grams fat, 1 gram protein

3. RANCH DIP

Ingredients:

- Ranch seasoning, two tablespoons
- Sour cream, one half cup
- Mayonnaise, one cup

Instructions

Mix all of the ingredients together and allow to chill for at least one hour before serving.

Nutrition info one quarter cup:

Calories 241, 1-gram net carbs, 26 grams fat, 1 gram protein

4. AVOCADO SAUCE

Ingredients:

- Pistachio nuts, two ounces
- Salt, one teaspoon
- Lime juice, one quarter cup
- Garlic, minced, two tablespoons
- Water, one quarter cup
- Olive oil, two-thirds cup
- Avocado, one
- Parsley or cilantro, fresh, one cup

Instructions

Use a food processor or a blender to mix all of the ingredients together until they are smooth except the pistachio nuts and olive oil. Ad these at the end and mix well. If the mix is a bit thick add in a bit more oil or water. This sauce will stay fresh in the refrigerator for up to four days.

Nutrition info per quarter cup:

Calories 490, 5 grams net carbs, 50 grams fat, 5 grams protein

5. BLUE CHEESE DRESSING

Ingredients:

- Parsley, fresh, two tablespoons
- Black pepper, one teaspoon
- Salt, one teaspoon
- Heavy whipping cream, one half cup
- Mayonnaise, one half cup
- Greek yogurt, three-fourths cup
- Blue cheese, five ounces

Instructions

Break the blue cheese up into small chunks in a large bowl. Stir in the heavy cream, mayonnaise, and yogurt. Mix in the parsley, salt, and pepper and let the dressing sit for one hour, so the flavors mix well. This dressing will be good in the refrigerator for three days.

Nutrition per one quarter cup:

Calories 477, 4 grams net carbs, 47 grams fat, 10 grams protein

6. SALSA DRESSING

Ingredients:

- Garlic, minced, one tablespoon
- Chili powder, one teaspoon
- Apple cider vinegar, three tablespoons
- Mayonnaise, two tablespoons
- Sour cream, two tablespoons
- Olive oil, one quarter cup
- Salsa, one half cup

Instructions

Add all of the ingredients to a large bowl and mix well. Pour into a glass jar and let the dressing chill in the refrigerator for at least one hour. This dressing will stay good in the refrigerator for three days.

Nutrition per one quarter cup:

Calories 200, 2 grams net carbs, 21 grams fat, 1-gram protein

7. GUACAMOLE

Ingredients:

- Salt, one half teaspoon
- Black pepper, one teaspoon
- Garlic, minced, one tablespoon
- Cilantro, four tablespoons
- Olive oil, two tablespoons
- Tomato, one diced small
- Lime juice, two tablespoons
- White onion, one half chopped finely
- Avocado, two ripe

Instructions

Wash, peel, and pit the avocados and mash the pulp with a fork. Stir in the garlic, salt, pepper, cilantro, olive oil, tomato, lime juice, and onion. Let the guacamole sit for at least two hours before serving.

Nutrition info one quarter cup:

Calories 238, 5 grams net carbs, 22 grams fat, 3 grams protein

8. SPICY PIMIENTO CHEESE

Ingredients:

- Cheddar cheese, shredded, one half cup
- Cayenne pepper, one eighth teaspoon
- Dijon mustard, one tablespoon
- Paprika, one teaspoon
- Chili powder, one teaspoon
- Pimientos, finely chopped, four tablespoons
- Mayonnaise, one third cup

Instructions

Cream all of the ingredients together and then refrigerate for at least one hour before serving. This cheese will stay good in the refrigerator for up to five days.

Nutrition info one quarter cup:

Calories 248, 1 gram net carbs, 24 grams fat, 7 grams protein

9. CAESAR DRESSING

Ingredients:

- Lemon juice, one tablespoon
- Anchovies, one ounce
- Salt, one half teaspoon
- Garlic, minced, one teaspoon
- Black pepper, one quarter teaspoon
- Apple cider vinegar, one teaspoon
- Dijon mustard, one tablespoon
- Olive oil, one half cup
- Parmesan cheese, grated, one quarter cup

Instructions

Blend together all of the ingredients. If the dressing seems to be a little too thick then add drops of water until it is the right consistency. This dressing will stay good in the refrigerator for up to three days.

Nutrition info per one quarter cup:

Calories 298, 1 gram net carbs, 31 grams fat, 6 grams protein

10. HUMMUS

Ingredients:

- Black pepper, one half teaspoon
- Salt, one half teaspoon
- Cumin, ground, one half teaspoon
- Garlic, minced, one tablespoon
- Lemon juice, two tablespoons
- Tahini, one quarter cup
- Sunflower seeds, one quarter cup
- Olive oil, one half cup
- Cilantro, fresh chopped, one half cup
- Avocados, three ripe

Instructions

Wash, dry, and peel the avocados. Take out the pits and drop the flesh into a food processor or a blender with the remainder of the ingredients. Mix everything well until the mix is smooth and creamy.

Nutrition info per quarter cup:

Calories 417, 4 grams net carbs, 41 grams fat, 5 grams protein

Chapter Eleven

SEVEN DAY MEAL PLAN

This is a sample seven-day meal plan for you to follow. This is only a suggestion and you should feel free to substitute any of the menu ideas for other menu items. All of these recipes are found in this book.

DAY ONE	
Breakfast	Cauliflower Hash Browns
Lunch	Pepperoni Pizza
Dinner	Tuna Casserole
DAY TWO	
Breakfast	Smoked Salmon Sandwich
Lunch	Tex Mex Stuffed Zucchini Boats
Dinner	Avocado Shrimp Boats
DAY THREE	
Breakfast	Coconut Porridge
Lunch	Deviled Egg Salad
Dinner	Bacon Wrapped Meatloaf
DAY FOUR	
Breakfast	Oatmeal
Lunch	Sloppy Joes
Dinner	White Fish with Curry and Coconut

DAY FIVE	
Breakfast	Scrambled Eggs with Halloumi Cheese
Lunch	Baked Fish Sticks
Dinner	Herbed Grilled Chicken
DAY SIX	
Breakfast	Mushroom Omelet
Lunch	Chicken Cabbage and Onions
Dinner	Spinach and Goat Cheese Pie
DAY SEVEN	
Breakfast	Coconut Cream with Berries
Lunch	Pigs in a Blanket
Dinner	Chicken Bacon Ranch Casserole

Chapter Twelve

SPICES FOR KETO COOKING

Your keto cooking will never be boring if you learn to use spices to flavor your food. Here is a list of common spices that you can experiment with to add in some flavor to the dishes you create.

Allspice: This single spice gives the flavor of cinnamon, nutmeg and cloves. It is usually used ground in recipes for poultry, seafood and meat marinades.

Basil: The sweet yet peppery taste of basil in used in pesto and almost always in any dish that contains tomatoes. Basil also works well with rosemary, parsley, thyme, oregano, and sage.

Bay Leaves: Potently flavored, just a leaf or two of bay will usually suffice in marinades for meats and poultry. It's even found in an occasional dessert.

Chives: These are a part of the onion family but they are milder and more delicate in flavor. They work well in salads and egg dishes.

Cilantro: A strongly aromatic seasoning that has a pungent flavor reminiscent of sage and lemon.

Cinnamon: This adds a warm spiciness to food. It complements meats and vegetables like carrots, spinach, and onions. Cinnamon is often used with other warm spices, like allspice, ginger, cardamom, nutmeg, cloves and pepper.

Cloves: Cloves are often used as a flavoring for meat dishes. This spice also works well with black pepper, ginger, nutmeg, and cinnamon.

Coriander: This spice is often used to flavor meat, poultry, and vegetable dishes. It has an orangey scent and tastes sweet and warm.

Cumin: This spice works well in recipes for eggs, seafood, meats and poultry, as well as sauces that are tomato based.

Garlic: This is a versatile seasoning that complements most any savory dish. Garlic can be used to flavor almost any dish.

Ginger: This spice works well in sauces and stir fries, especially any dish with an Asian flair.

Marjoram: This is a relative of oregano with but with a lighter, more delicate flavor. It works well with many vegetables, poultry and meats.

Nutmeg: This spice is used in recipes for seafood, poultry, eggs, cheeses, and vegetables (especially eggplant, spinach, and cabbage).

Onion: These come in many varieties and sizes and can be used anywhere you want to use them.

Oregano: Oregano is related to marjoram, but its flavor is stronger. You will usually find it in tomato-based recipes. It pairs up well with other spices, like thyme, garlic, basil, and parsley.

Paprika: This spice is used in vegetable dishes as well as eggs and poultry. It is especially useful as a garnish due to its beautiful color.

Parsley: Parsley is used in meat marinades, dressings, salads, casseroles, and omelets.

Pepper: This spice comes in ground black pepper and the lighter flavored ground white pepper.

Rosemary: This spice is used liberally in marinades and with roasted and grilled foods, like vegetables, poultry, and seafood.

Sage: Sage has a pungent, slightly bitter/sweet taste and an herbal fragrance. It is especially good in meats, seafood, poultry, and dressings.

Thyme: This is a pungent seasoning that has a minty flavor and scent. Try it, lightly in the beginning, with meat, seafood, poultry, and in marinades.

Conclusion

Thank you for making it through to the end of *Keto for Women Over 50*, let's hope it was informative and able to provide you with all of the tools you need to achieve your goals whatever they may be.

The next step is to make the commitment to follow the keto lifestyle and begin your journey to a new and better life. While you might be a woman over 50 you still have a lot of life to live and you should be able to live that life to the fullest. And that will begin with the best possible nutrition that will give you the health and the ability to be active that will carry you into the next phase of your life.

Finally, if you found this book useful in any way, a review on Amazon is always appreciated!

Made in the USA
Middletown, DE
12 January 2020